# DEAR DAD, CAN WE TALK ABOUT YOUR MEMORY?

Wisdom on Brain Health

# DEAR DAD, CAN WE TALK ABOUT YOUR MEMORY?

## Wisdom on Brain Health

## Tara Rose, PhD

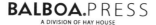

BALBOA.PRESS
A DIVISION OF HAY HOUSE

Balboa Press books may be ordered through booksellers or by contacting:

Balboa Press
A Division of Hay House
1663 Liberty Drive
Bloomington, IN 47403
www.balboapress.com
1 (877) 407-4847

Print information available on the last page.

ISBN: 978-1-9822-3993-0 (sc)
ISBN: 978-1-9822-3994-7 (e)

Library of Congress Control Number: 2019920765

Balboa Press rev. date: 12/19/2019

This book is dedicated to my father, Mel Martin.

May his memory be a blessing always.

# Contents

Hindi-language

# Introduction

This is a Dear Dad letter.

I wrote to my dad after visiting him because he was having some memory problems.  The problems were not very severe, but he noticed them, and we were concerned.  It is a letter of love from a daughter to her father, quite informal in tone, and also containing detailed information that is not typical for such a correspondence.  My father and I spent much of our careers  working in hospitals. I have an area of expertise in education about dementia and Alzheimer's, and so naturally I wanted him to know the latest in research.

While I wrote this letter for my dad, I never did give it to him – he passed a couple of months later (not related to his memory problems).  When I first began to share this letter and the worksheets "Am I having memory problems?" and "Am I taking care of my brain health?", it seemed like way to honor my Dad. It's now been over three years and I've updated the information while retaining my original daughter's voice speaking to my father.

I wanted to give that background and a warning to the reader because the letter is a bit detailed at times, so I thought it might be helpful to know something about my father and myself. My dad was a retired pharmacist and hospital senior administrator.  I am a clinical psychologist specializing in gerontology, working at the Alzheimer's Disease Research Center (ADRC) at the University of Southern California funded by the National Institutes of Health (NIH).  As a result, the letter is written for someone who has a certain level of understanding of medical issues, broadly speaking.  I wanted to pass the information on to him, and now on to you.

# DEAR DAD, CAN WE TALK ABOUT YOUR MEMORY?

If there is something you don't understand, just skip over it for now, and you can always ask your doctor or health care provider about it later.

Please give this book to a parent, as you see appropriate. It can also go to a cousin, uncle, aunt, spouse, or friend.

You are welcome to use the information in this letter but please keep in mind that it is very important to go to a doctor if you are having memory problems. Please take this letter and your filled-out journal and bring it your physician or primary care provider. Do not take the contents of this letter as medical advice, but do read it carefully and take care of yourself. Significant memory problems are not a normal part of aging and there are many ways to reverse memory symptoms, protect yourself from dementia, and delay serious memory problems if you do have a disease.

Take care and be well,

Tara Rose

# Can We Talk About Your Memory?

Dear Dad,

You said you were having memory problems and have some questions. I thought it might be easiest to give you some advice you if I wrote it out in a letter. You know I research memory problems and that I have a lot of advice. And being your daughter, I think it is good advice. So just hear it, and know it comes from my heart. At the same time, is very academically focused, which has its limitations, but it seems like 30 years of Alzheimer's disease research might be a good starting place.

Let me start with the label of "memory problems." You asked me what the doctor will do if he determines that your level of memory issues is a problem. It's possible he would say that you have "mild cognitive impairment" (MCI). I know that many people worry about getting Alzheimer's disease or dementia as they get older. However, this letter is not about Alzheimer's disease or dementia, and let's not jump to conclusions simply because you are having some memory problems. Instead, I wanted to talk to you about what having some memory problems or MCI actually means. And so, let me tell you what the medical field and researchers are currently saying about MCI so that you can know about the latest research, have the information, and maybe get some relief by knowing the facts that will help you move forward.

Let me begin with an overview of what we currently know about mild memory problems.

Mild cognitive impairment (MCI) means that you are having noticeable changes in your memory and thinking. You have told me you have those symptoms but that they are not severe or serious enough to require help in your usual everyday activities. Sometimes this level of memory

3

problems is also called "mild neurocognitive disorder" (mNCD) which is defined as a noticeable change in cognitive functioning that goes beyond normal changes seen in aging. Remember: this is not dementia or Alzheimer's disease!

Before I go any further, I have to tell you what dementia and Alzheimer's Disease are so that you know why we are not talking about you having either of those very serious problems.

Dementia (occasionally called senility) means that someone is having significant memory problems. Dementia involves the loss of thinking, remembering, and reasoning (cognitive functioning) and ability to complete everyday tasks (behavioral abilities) to such an extent that it interferes with a person's daily life and activities. Dementia ranges in severity from the mildest stage, when it is just beginning to seriously affect a person's day-to-day functioning, to the most serious stage, when the person must depend completely on others for basic activities of daily living.

Alzheimer's disease is one of one of the main causes of dementia, but not the only cause. Alzheimer's disease is characterized by "plaques and tangles." Plaques are the build-up of proteins clusters and tangles are when important cells start to twist, and eventually die in the brain. So, a diagnosis of dementia means there are symptoms of serious memory loss. Alzheimer's disease is one of the possible causes of dementia, but not the only possible cause. In fact, there are multiple diseases that can cause dementia.

**The diagnosis of Dementia or Alzheimer's disease is a more severe situation than MCI (mild cognitive impairment).**

I'm trying to be reassuring here, I'm not sure how well I am doing… Here is a visual:

**Levels of Memory Problems:**

• **First, REGULAR memory problems as we age**

• **Second, BIGGER memory problems called Mild Cognitive Impairment (MCI)**

• **Third, SERIOUS memory problems called dementia or Alzheimer's disease**

That's it.

## Diagnosis, Treatment, Prognosis

Let me tell you what we (clinicians and researchers) know about mild cognitive impairment (MCI): the diagnosis, treatment, and longer-term prognosis of the kind of memory problems you might be having right now.

Overall, we can say that the 10% to 20% of people who are 65 years or older have MCI or mNCD.   We know that the risk of getting these problems increases with age, and that men appear to be at higher risk than women.

So, even though people with MCI are at greater risk for developing dementia compared with everyone else in the United States, there is quite a big range of risk estimates (from <5% to 20% annual conversion rates), depending on the group of people or population studied.  If someone has an MCI diagnosis, the chance each year of receiving a dementia diagnosis ranges from less than 5% to a 20% chance.  This means some people get better, some people stay the same, and some people's memory abilities do get worse.  As your daughter, I obviously wish for your memory to get better. There are many things that might be affecting your memory so let's get take action to get you corrected back to your "regular" memory.

There are a number of reasons that seniors can have MCI or increased risk for memory and thinking problems and other problems, including feeling sad or depressed (depression), multiple medications interacting with each other (polypharmacy), and problems with heart and blood flow in the body (uncontrolled cardiovascular risk factors). These things need to be looked into and considered by your doctor or primary care provider.

So, Dad, if you don't take care of whatever the situation is right now, and your memory concerns are reversible - you can actually cause permanent damage in some situations - so please take care of yourself and see your doctor right away!

As you can see, the big message of this letter is to see your doctor! And to take care of yourself, your well-being, and your health. Right now. I would like to tell you how you can start to take care of your health and memory and what to keep in mind when you see your doctor.

## WHAT CAN HELP RIGHT NOW? Take Care of YOURSELF!!

What can help you the most, and decrease your risk of memory problems?

First things first, take care of your body and your brain. They are connected, as you know. Taking care of ourselves can actually create positive physical changes in the brain. It's really amazing and the research is only a few years old. There is a lot of new research on how specific healthy habits (from the clinical trial studies) can change brain and improve brain functioning. They can actually see and measure the changes in the brain by scanning people's brains before they start the research study, then conducting the intervention with the new activity/habit, and then when the study is complete, scanning people's brains again. Researchers can now see that important areas of the brain actually grow or get healthier. It's like if you worked out and lifted weights, you would see your arm or leg muscles grow and get stronger.  Same thing for your brain. The difference is that we can't actually look inside the brain to see the changes, unless we use imaging that can be expensive. Because it can take time for our memories to improve, it can be easy to give up. But when we see that when our memory is better with time, it becomes worth establishing new habits and sticking to them.

I'm not going to write a lot on each topic on the following list because there are plenty of books out there.  I just want you to know which areas of basic keeping yourself healthy/being healthier are supported by research.  I know it takes a lot of effort to change these things and add new activities to our lives. There are areas that I could work on, too, so maybe we can do some of it together, even though we are not in the same city.

**1) Eat healthfully and drink enough water.**  Eat foods that are good for your heart.  You can look up "heart healthy" foods on the Internet.  Fruits and vegetables, whole grains, nuts, lean meats, and fish. There is a lot of talk about the "Mediterranean diet" which you can find online very quickly. Some studies have found specific vitamins and nutrients can improve health, and I will update you as more research comes out.  Right now, I can say getting enough Omega-3s is important and getting it from oily fish seems to be the best source.  That includes fatty fish like salmon, mackerel, and sardines.  There isn't any research that I know about yet on organic versus non-organic food, but since you are having memory problems, I think you should spend the extra money for organic food (food grown without pesticides or additives) as much as possible.  You/we are lucky enough to be able to afford the extra expense, and given that your brain is saying it needs help, please don't add chemicals that might be harmful to the body.

I also want to bring up another area that doesn't have enough research, which is taking a good multi-vitamin and supplements (as your provider recommends them).  Please take them.  It just seems that even if we don't have the research at this point, a body needs every advantage it can get to support memory.

Drinking enough water and staying hydrated is important. Dehydration can cause memory problems.

**2) Exercise.** Assuming your doctor says it is okay to exercise, make an exercise plan that includes cardio activities that get your heart rate up and also other activities for strength training. Exercise is the most amazing area for benefits, and wonderful new research using brain imaging actually shows change to the structure the brain, not just to the heart and muscles.

**3) Get plenty of sleep.** If you are not getting enough sleep, read about all the ways to sleep better or talk to your care provider. I love the analogy that describes sleep as when the garbage truck comes and picks up the trash in your brain that shouldn't be there. Don't cancel the trash removal service by skipping on sleep. Recent research studies confirm the benefits of sleep for brain health and well-being.

**4) Spend time with friends and family**. Socialize and talk to others. Have conversations with other people. Studies show that social activity is related to lower rates of memory decline, meaning your memory stays better longer. Researchers have shown that people who have more contact with people do better on tests of memory.

**5) Engage in risk reduction.** Risk reduction means to stop doing things we know are bad for our body and not good for our hearts. Smoking is a good example. We know this is bad for our overall health, and it can actually affect our brain, too.

A healthy heart is really important for our brains. It makes sense. We need the blood to get from the heart to the brain, so we need a healthy heart. And the blood caries the glucose or blood sugar to the brain, too – it is the energy for the brain. So, if someone has the wrong blood sugar going to the brain, too high too low or all over the place, it can wreak havoc in the brain and cause memory problems.

**A. Stop smoking.**  If you are smoking again, please stop.  Also, don't be around anyone who is smoking, because secondhand smoke is damaging, too.

**B. Diabetes.**  Have you had your blood sugar checked?  Diabetes, and even pre-diabetes (when the blood sugar levels are going up and down, and not regulated) is linked to dementia.  Cut down on the processed sugar, too, please.

**C. High blood pressure or hypertension.**  Controlling your blood pressure is really important.  Think about it – having unnecessary pressure on the brain  just doesn't sound good for us.

**D. Depression and anxiety.**  Research shows that people who have depression and anxiety are more likely to have memory problems.  We don't know for sure why, but it means getting some help addressing those feelings.  There are lots of treatments and approaches to help with depression and anxiety if you are experiencing this right now.

**E. Inflammation.**  Inflammation is not good for us. Inflammation of the blood brain barrier, the connection between the brain and a part of the neck or spine is especially bad.  If the blood brain barrier, that little "gate" where spinal fluid goes into the brain, is inflamed, it opens a little bit more, allowing other things to get into the brain and again wreak havoc. This means taking care of your body, including going to the dentist to avoid gum disease (which is a type of inflammation in the body).

**6. Exercise your brain.**  It's true that just like our body needs exercise, so does our brain.  Give your mind mentally challenging activities. It can be whatever you like.  Playing games, doing puzzles, reading, learning new things, having a hobby.  It could also be volunteering to help others, finding something meaningful to do with your time, especially in retirement.

**7. Reduce stress.** Chronic stress can actually damage the brain, making learning more difficult and causing memory problems. Meditation, yoga, and other mind-body activities have been shown to improve a lot of different problems. Meditation and yoga can even change our brains structure and reduce inflammation in areas of brain involved in memory.

**8. Music**. You love music so much, so listen to your favorite tunes or sing. I think it will make you happier and some new research shows that music stimulates different parts of the brain.

**9. Love and have gratitude.** Pray and be thankful. You taught me that so can I say it back to you now? Sit and breathe, be with God, however you do that. I'm not sure of the research on this last point, but I can't imagine any better advice.

These are a lot of ideas for brain health. Pick what works for you right now.

**See a Doctor or Health Care Provider**

Okay, now let's talk about going to the doctor or care provider to check out your memory problems. This is very important. I am going to be technical in this section, but since we both have worked at hospitals, I think you would rather have more details that can be helpful. If you are not sure about my points, then please ask your doctor to explain it to you.

**For the Appointment**

Be sure to **bring someone with you** to the doctor's appointment.

This is important advice. It will help if you can take someone close to you, who knows you well (like mom), who can confirm your memory concerns and give the message that you want the doctor to take your concerns seriously. Mom (or whoever you bring) can also take notes so you can just listen to the doctor.

**What does the doctor need to check if you are having memory problems or MCI?**

The doctor needs to have an understanding of the following aspects of your life: (You can help by making notes and a list before you go to your appointment.)

1. Changes in memory/cognitive function (when it started, how it has changed, examples of memory problems).

2. Changes in ability to do everyday activities. This includes activities of daily living, or how you manage your day and the difficulties you might be having including taking care of finances and money management.

3. Are you eating well and what about your drinking? Yes, both water and alcohol! Remember that being dehydrated (not drinking enough water) can cause memory problems.

4. Current prescriptions and over-the-counter medications. This includes vitamins and nutritional supplements.

5. Symptoms that might be related to the brain such as hearing, vision, speech, sleep problems, walking, numbness, or tingling in any part of the body.

6. Symptoms that are related to heart health – meaning that the brain gets enough and the right flow of blood from the heart to the brain and then it gets the right amount of blood sugar/glucose to the brain. I mentioned this earlier, so, if you have any symptoms such as high blood pressure, pre-diabetes or diabetes, or any heart problems including irregular heartbeat, prepare to discuss these with the physician.

7. Mental health or well-being issues such as depression, anxiety, behavior or personality changes that can cause memory problems.

8. Family history. The doctor will also want to know about our family history. As far as I know, we are lucky and don't have a family history of serious memory loss or dementia. Dad, if you know something different about the family, please tell the doctor.

**The physician or provider will want to perform a physical and also may want to give you a neurological examination.** I want the doctor to have a chance to ask you questions and perform a physical exam to see what is going on.

**Laboratory Blood Tests**

Ask for lab work or laboratory testing that is normal for your age because your memory concerns could be a condition caused by a vitamin or mineral deficiency.

This is what I know you should ask to be tested, at least if you have health insurance: Blood work includes a full metabolic panel, it needs to include: complete blood count, electrolytes, glucose, calcium, thyroid function, iron, vitamin B12, and folate. Your doctor may want to test other aspects of your blood and functioning.

The reason we want all these tests run on your blood is to identify possibly reversible forms of MCI including infection, renal problems, too little or too much magnesium, too little or too much calcium, blood glucose/sugar level problems (hyperglycemia), thyroid problems, and vitamin or nutrient problems (vitamin B12, iron, or folate deficiency). It wouldn't be a surprise to know you have something on this list given our American eating habits.

Additional laboratory testing can check renal function and liver function. Also, Lyme disease, syphilis, and HIV can reveal rarer causes for cognitive impairment. But just know, the physician may not start with these tests or ever test for the sexually transmitted diseases unless you say something.

There is also laboratory testing for sleep apnea, when people snore or have trouble breathing regularly at night. Sleep apnea can affect people's ability to concentrate and their memory ability during the day.

**Professional Medication Review: Why?**

You want a professional medication review. You know this since you are a pharmacist, and it's particularly important for people with memory concerns. Certain classes and combinations of medications can contribute to memory problems and cognitive impairment so all current prescriptions, over-the-counter medications, and vitamins should be reviewed.

You probably don't really need to know this now, but drug classes most likely to contribute to cognitive impairment include anticholinergics, opiates, benzodiazepines and nonbenzodiazepine hypnotics (e.g., zolpidem), digoxin, antihistamines, tricyclic antidepressants, skeletal muscle relaxants, and antiepileptics. Hormonal therapy (estrogen alone or estrogen plus progestin) for menopause has been shown to increase risk for the combined end point of MCI or dementia (not that it really applies to you, but you might find it interesting). In addition, hypotensives used to treat of hypertension (high blood pressure), hypertension, and then blood sugar problems including hypoglycemia, hyperglycemia, pre-diabetes (high blood sugar results), and diabetes may also contribute to cognitive problems.

**Memory or Cognitive Testing**

We want someone to do memory or cognitive testing with you. The health care professional will also do very basic memory or cognitive testing which takes from 10-20 minutes. There are a number of different tests the physician may use and he or she might include a test called the Montreal Cognitive Assessment (MoCA), the Mini-Cognitive Assessment Instrument

(Mini-Cog), or my favorite, the Modified Mini-Mental State test (3MS). If the physician wants to do more tests, just be glad that you are getting an even better and more comprehensive assessment. It will be helpful to have those results. And if the doctor talks with you again six months or a year from now, you will be able to see how your memory changed or stayed the same. Your very first memory test is called a "baseline" and again, it is very helpful to have done.

**Ask for Brain Scans: Imaging of Your Brain**

Technology is amazing and if it seems you are having memory problems, your doctor may order some brain scans – or images of your brain. Please say "yes" to this. It's painless, you just have to lie still for 30 - 45 minutes in a machine, and they take images of your brain.

There are a couple of different kinds of tests that create images of your brain. An MRI (Magnetic Resonance Imaging) or CT scans (Computerized Tomography, also called CAT Scan stands for Computerized Axial Tomography) are both good tests to have. Usually the doctor only orders one, or more.

Why do they do these kinds of brain scans? To look and see if there is any mass, hemorrhage, or infection. Since all of our brains shrink, the doctors also look at the "global mass volume" to see that the loss or shrinkage is consistent with your age, and not more than that. They also look for other kinds of brain or structural changes to make sure there is nothing unusual.

It is good to have these and other tests as a "baseline" as I mentioned earlier, and if you still have memory problems in a year or two and they don't resolve on their own, the doctor can have another scan done and then they can compare the results.

Another good reason to have the imaging, **is if you have had a stroke, a silent stoke (meaning one you don't know about) or a transient ischemic attack (TIA),** you may experience memory loss but may recover some or almost all of your previous functioning and memory. Often the residue of these strokes can be seen on the brain imaging technology which is important because you would want to see a cardiologist or neurologist to reduce or stop having these health problems – and make sure you don't have one again!

## What Do We Find out from the Assessment and Tests Results?

If any of the results or factors are significant, the doctor will try to treat those symptoms to see if your memory improves. The physician will also want to discuss what was found regarding an MCI diagnosis with both you and other family members (or whoever goes with you to the appointment).

Either way, the physician will want to see you again in six months. It is important to arrange for a follow-up appointment approximately every six months so the doctor can watch for changes (including improvements) in memory / cognitive function and also in your needs.

## Referral, If Needed Please

If you have any serious problems with your memory, I want the primary care physician/health care professional to refer you to a specialist. Experts are important and they know what to test for and also what can be helpful for you. This person is usually a neurologist or geriatric specialist (someone who works with older adults).

## Mild Cognitive Impairment Diagnosis

## What criteria are used for Diagnosing MCI?

Here is the information the doctor uses to diagnosis Mild Cognitive Impairment (MCI), but keep in mind that criteria may change:

1. Concern regarding a change in thinking abilities (cognition) from the person, from someone who knows the person or from a clinician observing the person.

2. "Objective evidence" of impairment (see testing above) in one or more cognitive area including memory, executive function, attention, language, or visuospatial skills.

3. Preservation of independence in functional abilities (although a person may be less efficient and make more errors at performing activities of daily living and instrumental activities of daily living than in the past).

4. No evidence of a significant impairment in social or occupational functioning (i.e., not having dementia).

I hope you can see this list shows some problems, but not severe problems, which is what mild cognitive impairment is labeled right now.

That is about it for details and what primary care providers or physicians can do to help you. Now I want to talk to you about some other things you can do once you leave the doctor's office to potentially help your memory.

**Please make an appointment with your primary care physician/general practitioner, and if you want, use the 10-week journal and worksheets below and bring them to the physician.**

You could fill out the journal and worksheets yourself, but sometimes other people who are close to you are better able to do this. Maybe Mom can fill it out for you, or we could do it over the phone. Let me know.

**I hope you are finding this helpful. I realize this is a long letter, but I wanted you to have the information since this is my field. I'm around, just call.**

**I love you, Dad. You are in my prayers, and may God give you health and well-being and peace.**

Love and more love,

Tara Rose

# Am I Having Memory Problems or Is This Normal?

# Worksheet

Fill out this form before going to your doctor or health care provider's office. Bring it with you to your health care appointment.

Your name:

_____

Doctor/Health Care Provider:

_____

Appointment Date:

_____

Doctor's/Provider's Phone Number:

_____

**I have concerns about my memory. I've written some notes and filled out this form about my memory concerns. Would you like me to read my notes? You can make a copy if you like.**

**MEMORY: I am concerned about these things and I would like to know if this is normal or not:**

I am concerned about my memory, when I:_____

_____

# DEAR DAD, CAN WE TALK ABOUT YOUR MEMORY?

I am also concerned about my memory, when I: _____

_____

Another memory concern I have is: _____

_____

Does anything make the memory problems worse or better? Are the memory concerns all the time or just sometimes (and when)?

    1. _____

    2. _____

These memory concern affect my day-to-day life by:

    1. _____

    2. _____

Medications, other physical problems:

_____

Mental health or well-being problems:

☐ Anxious or Anxiety   ☐ Sadness or Depression

_____

Other problems in your life (short list) (changes or things/events that are stressful or not easy to deal with):

_____

_____

_____

Please check the best box for the questions below. Some of the following memory concerns are normal and some can be problems. Use this checklist of possible normal and not so normal memory issues so the doctor can get an idea of how serious your concerns are and where the problems might be.

| Never NO | Sometimes/ A little | All the time YES | Does this happen to you? | # |
|---|---|---|---|---|
| | | | Absent-mindedness. usually happens when I am not paying close attention to what I am doing. | A |
| | | | Occasionally forgetting where I placed things. | B |
| | | | I have been forgetting facts over time. | C |
| | | | I sometimes have a "tip of the tongue" memory slip that I remember later. | D |
| | | | I regularly have trouble remembering words. Sometimes I say the wrong words. | E |
| | | | Using reminders help me remember. | F |
| | | | Sometimes, even with reminders, I still forget appointments or important things. | G |
| | | | It's harder for me to/ I am not interested in grooming or taking care of myself – like showering/bathing, changing my clothes. | H |
| | | | My memory is affecting or makes me less interested in my work | I |

Am I having Memory Problems Worksheet from *Dear Dad, Can We Talk About Your Memory* by Tara Rose, PhD, © 2019. Permission to photocopy is granted with purchase of book, see copyright page.

| Never NO | Sometimes/ A little | All the time YES | Does this happen to you? | # |
|---|---|---|---|---|
| | | | My memory is affecting or makes me less interested in my hobbies. | J |
| | | | My memory is affecting or makes me less interested in being social with people. | K |
| | | | My memory is affecting or makes me less interested in being social with people. | L |
| | | | I get embarrassed by my memory issues, and then I don't want to be around people. | M |
| | | | When I talk, I often pause to remember words or memories. | N |
| | | | I have been forgetting recent events and things that happen. | O |
| | | | I often forget where I put things like keys or a phone. | P |
| | | | The people around me notice memory problems, but I don't see a problem. | Q |
| | | | I have mood swings, get upset or angry more easily than I used to. | R |
| | | | I act differently towards people than I used to. | S |
| | | | I sometimes have difficulty performing simple, routine tasks like paying bills. | T |
| | | | I have trouble getting dressed. | U |
| | | | I sometimes have trouble with my meals. | V |

| Never NO | Sometimes/ A little | All the time YES | Does this happen to you? | # |
|---|---|---|---|---|
|  |  |  | Trouble paying attention and understanding a TV show or book | W |
|  |  |  | Trouble keeping track of current events | X |
|  |  |  | Sometimes I get lost in places like a store or mall I've been many times. | Y |
|  |  |  | Sometimes I get lost getting to places I've been to many times. | Z |
|  |  |  | I find myself repeating the same conversation over and over. | AA |
|  |  |  | Other people tell me I repeat the same thing over and over. | BB |

**Here are some things you may want to say to your doctor/health care professional at your appointment:**

"Can you do a memory screening test for me? Either at this appointment or at another appointment? I hear it only takes 10-15 minutes and I would like to know if there is a possible problem."

"If it seems there might be a problem or a possible question about my memory, I would like some blood work to be done to make sure I don't have any causes of memory problems that are reversible, like a vitamin deficiency. Here is a letter my daughter wrote that lists the kinds of blood work that I may need."

"Can you also check my medications to make sure there aren't any interactions?"

---

DEAR DAD, CAN WE TALK ABOUT YOUR MEMORY?

# Am I Having Memory Problems

## A 10-Week Journal – Week 1

Week: ☐ 1   ☐ 2   ☐ 3   ☐ 4   ☐ 5   ☐ 6   ☐ 7   ☐ 8   ☐ 9   ☐ 10

Today's date is: _____

☐ Monday  ☐ Tuesday  ☐ Wednesday  ☐ Thursday  ☐ Friday

☐ Saturday  ☐ Sunday

Big and small activities of the week or day:

_____

## Keeping Track of What I Am Forgetting

**My Memory issues/Forgetfulness this week:**

Did I forget something or have concerns about my memory today?

☐ Yes          ☐ No          ☐ Maybe

**This week, did I forget or have trouble with:** *(check if you had problems)*

**Forgetfulness:**

☐ Names     ☐ Keys     ☐ Wallet/bag/money     ☐ Cell phone

☐ What I wanted to say   ☐ Something else important_____

**Location:**

☐ Forgot day of the week   ☐ Forgot where I was

---

Am I Having Memory Problems and Am I Taking Care of My Brain Health: A 10 Week Journal from *Dear Dad, Can We Talk About Your Memory* by Tara Rose, PhD, © 2019. Permission to photocopy is granted with purchase of book, see copyright page.

**Felt confused**:

☐ What was I about to do  ☐ How to do something I normally do

**Lost:**

☐ Couldn't remember how to get somewhere

**Basics**:

☐ Problem getting dressed      ☐ How to cook or get a meal

☐ How to pay a bill

**What did I have problems with?**

_____

☐ I had memory problems but I don't remember what they were

**Notes:**

Am I Having Memory Problems and Am I Taking Care of My Brain Health: A 10 Week Journal from
*Dear Dad, Can We Talk About Your Memory* by Tara Rose, PhD, © 2019. Permission to photocopy is granted
with purchase of book, see copyright page.

# Am I Taking Care of my Brain Health

# A 10-Week Journal – Week 1

Week: ☐ 1 ☐ 2 ☐ 3 ☐ 4 ☐ 5 ☐ 6 ☐ 7 ☐ 8 ☐ 9 ☐ 10

Today's date is: _____

☐ Monday ☐ Tuesday ☐ Wednesday ☐ Thursday ☐ Friday

☐ Saturday ☐ Sunday

Big and small activities of the week or day:

_____

# Keeping Track of Healthy Brain Health

**Brain Health:** ☐ **Today I:** ☐ **This week I:**

1. Drank enough water and made sure I was hydrated?

    ☐ Yes      ☐ No      ☐ Maybe/Somewhat

2. Ate healthy?

    ☐ Yes      ☐ No      ☐ Maybe/Somewhat

3. Took my medication and/or vitamins for the day?

    ☐ Yes      ☐ No      ☐ Maybe/Somewhat

4. Had enough / good sleep last night?

    ☐ Yes      ☐ No      ☐ Maybe/Somewhat

5. Had stress?

☐ Yes          ☐ No          ☐ Maybe/Somewhat

Managed the stress well?

☐ Yes          ☐ No          ☐ Maybe/Somewhat

6. Did body exercise (walk, aerobics, etc.)?

☐ Yes          ☐ No          ☐ Maybe/Somewhat

7. Had some kind of brain exercise?

☐ Yes          ☐ No          ☐ Maybe/Somewhat

8. Had social time / time with family or friends?

☐ Yes          ☐ No          ☐ Maybe/Somewhat

9. Other ways to take care of brain health?

_____

☐ Yes          ☐ No          ☐ Maybe/Somewhat

10. Other ways to take care of brain health?

_____

☐ Yes          ☐ No          ☐ Maybe/Somewhat

Notes:

# Am I Having Memory Problems

## A 10-Week Journal – Week 2

Week: ☐ 1  ☐ 2  ☐ 3  ☐ 4  ☐ 5  ☐ 6  ☐ 7  ☐ 8  ☐ 9  ☐ 10

Today's date is: _____

☐ Monday  ☐ Tuesday  ☐ Wednesday  ☐ Thursday  ☐ Friday

☐ Saturday  ☐ Sunday

Big and small activities of the week or day:

_____

## Keeping Track of What I Am Forgetting

**My Memory issues/Forgetfulness this week:**

Did I forget something or have concerns about my memory today?

☐ Yes          ☐ No          ☐ Maybe

**This week, did I forget or have trouble with:** *(check if you had problems)*

**Forgetfulness:**

☐ Names      ☐ Keys      ☐ Wallet/bag/money      ☐ Cell phone

☐ What I wanted to say      ☐ Something else important_____

**Location:**

☐ Forgot day of the week  ☐ Forgot where I was

---

Am I Having Memory Problems and Am I Taking Care of My Brain Health: A 10 Week Journal from *Dear Dad, Can We Talk About Your Memory* by Tara Rose, PhD, © 2019. Permission to photocopy is granted with purchase of book, see copyright page.

**Felt confused**:

☐ What was I about to do   ☐ How to do something I normally do

**Lost:**

☐ Couldn't remember how to get somewhere

**Basics**:

☐ Problem getting dressed       ☐ How to cook or get a meal

☐ How to pay a bill

**What did I have problems with?**

_____

☐ I had memory problems but I don't remember what they were

**Notes:**

# Am I Taking Care of my Brain Health

# A 10-Week Journal – Week 2

Week: ☐ 1  ☐ 2  ☐ 3  ☐ 4  ☐ 5  ☐ 6  ☐ 7  ☐ 8  ☐ 9  ☐ 10

Today's date is: _____

☐ Monday  ☐ Tuesday  ☐ Wednesday  ☐ Thursday  ☐ Friday

☐ Saturday  ☐ Sunday

Big and small activities of the week or day:

_____

# Keeping Track of Healthy Brain Health

**Brain Health:  ☐ Today I:   ☐ This week I:**

1. Drank enough water and made sure I was hydrated?

   ☐ Yes          ☐ No          ☐ Maybe/Somewhat

2. Ate healthy?

   ☐ Yes          ☐ No          ☐ Maybe/Somewhat

3. Took my medication and/or vitamins for the day?

   ☐ Yes          ☐ No          ☐ Maybe/Somewhat

4. Had enough / good sleep last night?

   ☐ Yes          ☐ No          ☐ Maybe/Somewhat

5. Had stress?

☐ Yes ☐ No ☐ Maybe/Somewhat

Managed the stress well?

☐ Yes ☐ No ☐ Maybe/Somewhat

6. Did body exercise (walk, aerobics, etc.)?

☐ Yes ☐ No ☐ Maybe/Somewhat

7. Had some kind of brain exercise?

☐ Yes ☐ No ☐ Maybe/Somewhat

8. Had social time / time with family or friends?

☐ Yes ☐ No ☐ Maybe/Somewhat

9. Other ways to take care of brain health?

_____

☐ Yes ☐ No ☐ Maybe/Somewhat

10. Other ways to take care of brain health?

_____

☐ Yes ☐ No ☐ Maybe/Somewhat

**Notes:**

# Am I Having Memory Problems
# A 10-Week Journal – Week 3

Week: □ 1  □ 2  □ 3  □ 4  □ 5  □ 6  □ 7  □ 8  □ 9  □ 10

Today's date is: _____

□ Monday  □ Tuesday  □ Wednesday  □ Thursday  □ Friday

□ Saturday  □ Sunday

Big and small activities of the week or day:

_____

# Keeping Track of What I Am Forgetting

**My Memory issues/Forgetfulness this week:**

Did I forget something or have concerns about my memory today?

□ Yes          □ No          □ Maybe

**This week, did I forget or have trouble with:** *(check if you had problems)*

**Forgetfulness:**

□ Names     □ Keys     □ Wallet/bag/money     □ Cell phone

□ What I wanted to say     □ Something else important_____

**Location:**

□ Forgot day of the week  □ Forgot where I was

---

**Felt confused**:

☐ What was I about to do ☐ How to do something I normally do

**Lost:**

☐ Couldn't remember how to get somewhere

**Basics**:

☐ Problem getting dressed ☐ How to cook or get a meal

☐ How to pay a bill

**What did I have problems with?**

_____

☐ I had memory problems but I don't remember what they were

**Notes:**

Am I Having Memory Problems and Am I Taking Care of My Brain Health: A 10 Week Journal from *Dear Dad, Can We Talk About Your Memory* by Tara Rose, PhD, © 2019. Permission to photocopy is granted with purchase of book, see copyright page.

# Am I Taking Care of my Brain Health

# A 10-Week Journal – Week 3

Week: ☐ 1   ☐ 2   ☐ 3   ☐ 4   ☐ 5   ☐ 6   ☐ 7   ☐ 8   ☐ 9   ☐ 10

Today's date is: _____

☐ Monday  ☐ Tuesday  ☐ Wednesday  ☐ Thursday  ☐ Friday

☐ Saturday  ☐ Sunday

Big and small activities of the week or day:

_____

# Keeping Track of Healthy Brain Health

**Brain Health:  ☐ Today I:   ☐ This week I:**

1. Drank enough water and made sure I was hydrated?

☐ Yes          ☐ No          ☐ Maybe/Somewhat

2. Ate healthy?

☐ Yes          ☐ No          ☐ Maybe/Somewhat

3. Took my medication and/or vitamins for the day?

☐ Yes          ☐ No          ☐ Maybe/Somewhat

4. Had enough / good sleep last night?

☐ Yes          ☐ No          ☐ Maybe/Somewhat

5. Had stress?

    ☐ Yes    ☐ No    ☐ Maybe/Somewhat

    Managed the stress well?

    ☐ Yes    ☐ No    ☐ Maybe/Somewhat

6. Did body exercise (walk, aerobics, etc.)?

    ☐ Yes    ☐ No    ☐ Maybe/Somewhat

7. Had some kind of brain exercise?

    ☐ Yes    ☐ No    ☐ Maybe/Somewhat

8. Had social time / time with family or friends?

    ☐ Yes    ☐ No    ☐ Maybe/Somewhat

9. Other ways to take care of brain health?

_____

    ☐ Yes    ☐ No    ☐ Maybe/Somewhat

10. Other ways to take care of brain health?

_____

    ☐ Yes    ☐ No    ☐ Maybe/Somewhat

**Notes:**

# Am I Having Memory Problems

## A 10-Week Journal – Week 4

Week: ☐ 1　☐ 2　☐ 3　☐ 4　☐ 5　☐ 6　☐ 7　☐ 8　☐ 9　☐ 10

Today's date is: _____

☐ Monday　☐ Tuesday　☐ Wednesday　☐ Thursday　☐ Friday

☐ Saturday　☐ Sunday

Big and small activities of the week or day:

_____

## Keeping Track of What I Am Forgetting

**My Memory issues/Forgetfulness this week:**

Did I forget something or have concerns about my memory today?

☐ Yes　　　☐ No　　　☐ Maybe

**This week, did I forget or have trouble with:** *(check if you had problems)*

**Forgetfulness:**

☐ Names　　☐ Keys　　☐ Wallet/bag/money　　☐ Cell phone

☐ What I wanted to say　　☐ Something else important_____

**Location:**

☐ Forgot day of the week　　☐ Forgot where I was

---

**Felt confused**:

☐ What was I about to do  ☐ How to do something I normally do

**Lost:**

☐ Couldn't remember how to get somewhere

**Basics**:

☐ Problem getting dressed    ☐ How to cook or get a meal

☐ How to pay a bill

**What did I have problems with?**

_____

☐ I had memory problems but I don't remember what they were


**Notes:**

# Am I Taking Care of my Brain Health?

## A 10-Week Journal – Week 4

Week: ☐ 1  ☐ 2  ☐ 3  ☐ 4  ☐ 5  ☐ 6  ☐ 7  ☐ 8  ☐ 9  ☐ 10

Today's date is: _____

☐ Monday  ☐ Tuesday  ☐ Wednesday ☐ Thursday ☐ Friday

☐ Saturday ☐ Sunday

Big and small activities of the week or day:

_____

## Keeping Track of Healthy Brain Health

**Brain Health:  ☐ Today I:  ☐ This week I:**

1. Drank enough water and made sure I was hydrated?

   ☐ Yes          ☐ No          ☐ Maybe/Somewhat

2. Ate healthy?

   ☐ Yes          ☐ No          ☐ Maybe/Somewhat

3. Took my medication and/or vitamins for the day?

   ☐ Yes          ☐ No          ☐ Maybe/Somewhat

4. Had enough / good sleep last night?

   ☐ Yes          ☐ No          ☐ Maybe/Somewhat

_____

5. Had stress?

☐ Yes       ☐ No       ☐ Maybe/Somewhat

Managed the stress well?

☐ Yes       ☐ No       ☐ Maybe/Somewhat

6. Did body exercise (walk, aerobics, etc.)?

☐ Yes       ☐ No       ☐ Maybe/Somewhat

7. Had some kind of brain exercise?

☐ Yes       ☐ No       ☐ Maybe/Somewhat

8. Had social time / time with family or friends?

☐ Yes       ☐ No       ☐ Maybe/Somewhat

9. Other ways to take care of brain health?

_____

☐ Yes       ☐ No       ☐ Maybe/Somewhat

10. Other ways to take care of brain health?

_____

☐ Yes       ☐ No       ☐ Maybe/Somewhat

**Notes:**

# Am I Having Memory Problems

## A 10-Week Journal – Week 5

Week: ☐ 1  ☐ 2  ☐ 3  ☐ 4  ☐ 5  ☐ 6  ☐ 7  ☐ 8  ☐ 9  ☐ 10

Today's date is: _____

☐ Monday  ☐ Tuesday  ☐ Wednesday  ☐ Thursday  ☐ Friday

☐ Saturday  ☐ Sunday

Big and small activities of the week or day:

_____

## Keeping Track of What I Am Forgetting

**My Memory issues/Forgetfulness this week:**

Did I forget something or have concerns about my memory today?

☐ Yes          ☐ No          ☐ Maybe

**This week, did I forget or have trouble with:** *(check if you had problems)*

**Forgetfulness:**

☐ Names      ☐ Keys      ☐ Wallet/bag/money      ☐ Cell phone

☐ What I wanted to say      ☐ Something else important_____

**Location:**

☐ Forgot day of the week  ☐ Forgot where I was

---

Am I Having Memory Problems and Am I Taking Care of My Brain Health: A 10 Week Journal from *Dear Dad, Can We Talk About Your Memory* by Tara Rose, PhD, © 2019. Permission to photocopy is granted with purchase of book, see copyright page.

**Felt confused**:

☐ What was I about to do  ☐ How to do something I normally do

**Lost:**

☐ Couldn't remember how to get somewhere

**Basics**:

☐ Problem getting dressed        ☐ How to cook or get a meal

☐ How to pay a bill

**What did I have problems with?**

_____

☐ I had memory problems but I don't remember what they were


**Notes:**

Am I Having Memory Problems and Am I Taking Care of My Brain Health: A 10 Week Journal from
*Dear Dad, Can We Talk About Your Memory* by Tara Rose, PhD, © 2019. Permission to photocopy is granted
with purchase of book, see copyright page.

# Am I Taking Care of my Brain Health?

# A 10-Week Journal – Week 5

Week: ☐ 1  ☐ 2  ☐ 3  ☐ 4  ☐ 5  ☐ 6  ☐ 7  ☐ 8  ☐ 9  ☐ 10

Today's date is: _____

☐ Monday  ☐ Tuesday  ☐ Wednesday  ☐ Thursday  ☐ Friday

☐ Saturday  ☐ Sunday

Big and small activities of the week or day:

_____

# Keeping Track of Healthy Brain Health

**Brain Health:  ☐ Today I:  ☐ This week I:**

1. Drank enough water and made sure I was hydrated?

    ☐ Yes        ☐ No        ☐ Maybe/Somewhat

2. Ate healthy?

    ☐ Yes        ☐ No        ☐ Maybe/Somewhat

3. Took my medication and/or vitamins for the day?

    ☐ Yes        ☐ No        ☐ Maybe/Somewhat

4. Had enough / good sleep last night?

    ☐ Yes        ☐ No        ☐ Maybe/Somewhat

5. Had stress?

☐ Yes   ☐ No   ☐ Maybe/Somewhat

Managed the stress well?

☐ Yes   ☐ No   ☐ Maybe/Somewhat

6. Did body exercise (walk, aerobics, etc.)?

☐ Yes   ☐ No   ☐ Maybe/Somewhat

7. Had some kind of brain exercise?

☐ Yes   ☐ No   ☐ Maybe/Somewhat

8. Had social time / time with family or friends?

☐ Yes   ☐ No   ☐ Maybe/Somewhat

9. Other ways to take care of brain health?

_____

☐ Yes   ☐ No   ☐ Maybe/Somewhat

10. Other ways to take care of brain health?

_____

☐ Yes   ☐ No   ☐ Maybe/Somewhat

**Notes:**

# Am I Having Memory Problems?

## A 10-Week Journal – Week 6

Week: ☐ 1 ☐ 2 ☐ 3 ☐ 4 ☐ 5 ☐ 6 ☐ 7 ☐ 8 ☐ 9 ☐ 10

Today's date is: _____

    ☐ Monday ☐ Tuesday ☐ Wednesday ☐ Thursday ☐ Friday

    ☐ Saturday ☐ Sunday

Big and small activities of the week or day:

_____

## Keeping Track of What I Am Forgetting

**My Memory issues/Forgetfulness this week:**

Did I forget something or have concerns about my memory today?

    ☐ Yes      ☐ No      ☐ Maybe

**This week, did I forget or have trouble with:** *(check if you had problems)*

**Forgetfulness:**

☐ Names     ☐ Keys     ☐ Wallet/bag/money     ☐ Cell phone

☐ What I wanted to say     ☐ Something else important_____

**Location:**

☐ Forgot day of the week     ☐ Forgot where I was

**Felt confused**:

☐ What was I about to do   ☐ How to do something I normally do

**Lost:**

☐ Couldn't remember how to get somewhere

**Basics**:

☐ Problem getting dressed        ☐ How to cook or get a meal

☐ How to pay a bill

**What did I have problems with?**

_____

☐ I had memory problems but I don't remember what they were

**Notes:**

Am I Having Memory Problems and Am I Taking Care of My Brain Health: A 10 Week Journal from *Dear Dad, Can We Talk About Your Memory* by Tara Rose, PhD, © 2019. Permission to photocopy is granted with purchase of book, see copyright page.

# Am I Taking Care of my Brain Health?

## A 10-Week Journal – Week 6

Week: ☐ 1  ☐ 2  ☐ 3  ☐ 4  ☐ 5  ☐ 6  ☐ 7  ☐ 8  ☐ 9  ☐ 10

Today's date is: _____

☐ Monday  ☐ Tuesday  ☐ Wednesday ☐ Thursday ☐ Friday

☐ Saturday ☐ Sunday

Big and small activities of the week or day:

---

## Keeping Track of Healthy Brain Health

**Brain Health:  ☐ Today I:  ☐ This week I:**

1. Drank enough water and made sure I was hydrated?

    ☐ Yes      ☐ No      ☐ Maybe/Somewhat

2. Ate healthy?

    ☐ Yes      ☐ No      ☐ Maybe/Somewhat

3. Took my medication and/or vitamins for the day?

    ☐ Yes      ☐ No      ☐ Maybe/Somewhat

4. Had enough / good sleep last night?

    ☐ Yes      ☐ No      ☐ Maybe/Somewhat

5. Had stress?

☐ Yes        ☐ No        ☐ Maybe/Somewhat

    Managed the stress well?

☐ Yes        ☐ No        ☐ Maybe/Somewhat

6. Did body exercise (walk, aerobics, etc.)?

☐ Yes        ☐ No        ☐ Maybe/Somewhat

7. Had some kind of brain exercise?

☐ Yes        ☐ No        ☐ Maybe/Somewhat

8. Had social time / time with family or friends?

☐ Yes        ☐ No        ☐ Maybe/Somewhat

9. Other ways to take care of brain health?

_____

☐ Yes        ☐ No        ☐ Maybe/Somewhat

10. Other ways to take care of brain health?

_____

☐ Yes        ☐ No        ☐ Maybe/Somewhat

**Notes:**

# Am I Having Memory Problems?

## A 10-Week Journal – Week 7

Week: ☐ 1  ☐ 2  ☐ 3  ☐ 4  ☐ 5  ☐ 6  ☐ 7  ☐ 8  ☐ 9  ☐ 10

Today's date is: _____

☐ Monday  ☐ Tuesday  ☐ Wednesday  ☐ Thursday  ☐ Friday

☐ Saturday  ☐ Sunday

Big and small activities of the week or day:

_____

## Keeping Track of What I Am Forgetting

**My Memory issues/Forgetfulness this week:**

Did I forget something or have concerns about my memory today?

☐ Yes          ☐ No          ☐ Maybe

**This week, did I forget or have trouble with:** *(check if you had problems)*

**Forgetfulness:**

☐ Names      ☐ Keys      ☐ Wallet/bag/money      ☐ Cell phone

☐ What I wanted to say      ☐ Something else important_____

**Location:**

☐ Forgot day of the week  ☐ Forgot where I was

---

Am I Having Memory Problems and Am I Taking Care of My Brain Health: A 10 Week Journal from *Dear Dad, Can We Talk About Your Memory* by Tara Rose, PhD, © 2019. Permission to photocopy is granted with purchase of book, see copyright page.

**Felt confused**:

☐ What was I about to do  ☐ How to do something I normally do

**Lost:**

☐ Couldn't remember how to get somewhere

**Basics**:

☐ Problem getting dressed  ☐ How to cook or get a meal

☐ How to pay a bill

**What did I have problems with?**

_____

☐ I had memory problems but I don't remember what they were

**Notes:**

# Am I Taking Care of my Brain Health?

## A 10-Week Journal – Week 7

Week: □ 1  □ 2  □ 3  □ 4  □ 5  □ 6  □ 7  □ 8  □ 9  □ 10

Today's date is: _____

□ Monday  □ Tuesday  □ Wednesday  □ Thursday  □ Friday

□ Saturday  □ Sunday

Big and small activities of the week or day:

_____

## Keeping Track of Healthy Brain Health

**Brain Health:  □ Today I:   □ This week I:**

1. Drank enough water and made sure I was hydrated?

    □ Yes          □ No          □ Maybe/Somewhat

2. Ate healthy?

    □ Yes          □ No          □ Maybe/Somewhat

3. Took my medication and/or vitamins for the day?

    □ Yes          □ No          □ Maybe/Somewhat

4. Had enough / good sleep last night?

    □ Yes          □ No          □ Maybe/Somewhat

_____

5. Had stress?

    ☐ Yes      ☐ No      ☐ Maybe/Somewhat

    Managed the stress well?

    ☐ Yes      ☐ No      ☐ Maybe/Somewhat

6. Did body exercise (walk, aerobics, etc.)?

    ☐ Yes      ☐ No      ☐ Maybe/Somewhat

7. Had some kind of brain exercise?

    ☐ Yes      ☐ No      ☐ Maybe/Somewhat

8. Had social time / time with family or friends?

    ☐ Yes      ☐ No      ☐ Maybe/Somewhat

9. Other ways to take care of brain health?

_____

    ☐ Yes      ☐ No      ☐ Maybe/Somewhat

10. Other ways to take care of brain health?

_____

    ☐ Yes      ☐ No      ☐ Maybe/Somewhat

**Notes:**

# Am I Having Memory Problems

## A 10-Week Journal – Week 8

Week: ☐ 1  ☐ 2  ☐ 3  ☐ 4  ☐ 5  ☐ 6  ☐ 7  ☐ 8  ☐ 9  ☐ 10

Today's date is: _____

☐ Monday  ☐ Tuesday  ☐ Wednesday  ☐ Thursday  ☐ Friday

☐ Saturday  ☐ Sunday

Big and small activities of the week or day:

_____

## Keeping Track of What I Am Forgetting

**My Memory issues/Forgetfulness this week:**

Did I forget something or have concerns about my memory today?

☐ Yes  ☐ No  ☐ Maybe

**This week, did I forget or have trouble with:** *(check if you had problems)*

**Forgetfulness:**

☐ Names  ☐ Keys  ☐ Wallet/bag/money  ☐ Cell phone

☐ What I wanted to say  ☐ Something else important_____

**Location:**

☐ Forgot day of the week  ☐ Forgot where I was

**Felt confused**:

☐ What was I about to do   ☐ How to do something I normally do

**Lost:**

☐ Couldn't remember how to get somewhere

**Basics**:

☐ Problem getting dressed       ☐ How to cook or get a meal

☐ How to pay a bill

**What did I have problems with?**

_____

☐ I had memory problems but I don't remember what they were

**Notes:**

# Am I Taking Care of my Brain Health?

## A 10-Week Journal – Week 8

Week: ☐ 1  ☐ 2  ☐ 3  ☐ 4  ☐ 5  ☐ 6  ☐ 7  ☐ 8  ☐ 9  ☐ 10

Today's date is: _____

☐ Monday  ☐ Tuesday  ☐ Wednesday  ☐ Thursday  ☐ Friday

☐ Saturday  ☐ Sunday

Big and small activities of the week or day:

_____

## Keeping Track of Healthy Brain Health

**Brain Health:  ☐ Today I:  ☐ This week I:**

1. Drank enough water and made sure I was hydrated?

  ☐ Yes          ☐ No          ☐ Maybe/Somewhat

2. Ate healthy?

  ☐ Yes          ☐ No          ☐ Maybe/Somewhat

3. Took my medication and/or vitamins for the day?

  ☐ Yes          ☐ No          ☐ Maybe/Somewhat

4. Had enough / good sleep last night?

  ☐ Yes          ☐ No          ☐ Maybe/Somewhat

5. Had stress?

☐ Yes      ☐ No      ☐ Maybe/Somewhat

Managed the stress well?

☐ Yes      ☐ No      ☐ Maybe/Somewhat

6. Did body exercise (walk, aerobics, etc.)?

☐ Yes      ☐ No      ☐ Maybe/Somewhat

7. Had some kind of brain exercise?

☐ Yes      ☐ No      ☐ Maybe/Somewhat

8. Had social time / time with family or friends?

☐ Yes      ☐ No      ☐ Maybe/Somewhat

9. Other ways to take care of brain health?

_____

☐ Yes      ☐ No      ☐ Maybe/Somewhat

10. Other ways to take care of brain health?

_____

☐ Yes      ☐ No      ☐ Maybe/Somewhat

**Notes:**

# Am I Having Memory Problems

## A 10-Week Journal – Week 9

Week: ☐ 1　☐ 2　☐ 3　☐ 4　☐ 5　☐ 6　☐ 7　☐ 8　☐ 9　☐ 10

Today's date is: _____

☐ Monday　☐ Tuesday　☐ Wednesday　☐ Thursday　☐ Friday

☐ Saturday　☐ Sunday

Big and small activities of the week or day:

_____

## Keeping Track of What I Am Forgetting

**My Memory issues/Forgetfulness this week:**

Did I forget something or have concerns about my memory today?

☐ Yes　　　☐ No　　　☐ Maybe

**This week, did I forget or have trouble with:** *(check if you had problems)*

**Forgetfulness:**

☐ Names　　☐ Keys　　☐ Wallet/bag/money　　☐ Cell phone

☐ What I wanted to say　　☐ Something else important_____

**Location:**

☐ Forgot day of the week　☐ Forgot where I was

**Felt confused**:

☐ What was I about to do ☐ How to do something I normally do

**Lost:**

☐ Couldn't remember how to get somewhere

**Basics**:

☐ Problem getting dressed    ☐ How to cook or get a meal

☐ How to pay a bill

**What did I have problems with?**

_____

☐ I had memory problems but I don't remember what they were

**Notes:**

# Am I Taking Care of my Brain Health?

## A 10-Week Journal – Week 9

Week: ☐ 1   ☐ 2   ☐ 3   ☐ 4   ☐ 5   ☐ 6   ☐ 7   ☐ 8   ☐ 9   ☐ 10

Today's date is: _____

☐ Monday  ☐ Tuesday  ☐ Wednesday  ☐ Thursday  ☐ Friday

☐ Saturday  ☐ Sunday

Big and small activities of the week or day:

---

## Keeping Track of Healthy Brain Health

**Brain Health:  ☐ Today I:   ☐ This week I:**

1. Drank enough water and made sure I was hydrated?

☐ Yes          ☐ No          ☐ Maybe/Somewhat

2. Ate healthy?

☐ Yes          ☐ No          ☐ Maybe/Somewhat

3. Took my medication and/or vitamins for the day?

☐ Yes          ☐ No          ☐ Maybe/Somewhat

4. Had enough / good sleep last night?

☐ Yes          ☐ No          ☐ Maybe/Somewhat

5. Had stress?

   ☐ Yes    ☐ No    ☐ Maybe/Somewhat

   Managed the stress well?

   ☐ Yes    ☐ No    ☐ Maybe/Somewhat

6. Did body exercise (walk, aerobics, etc.)?

   ☐ Yes    ☐ No    ☐ Maybe/Somewhat

7. Had some kind of brain exercise?

   ☐ Yes    ☐ No    ☐ Maybe/Somewhat

8. Had social time / time with family or friends?

   ☐ Yes    ☐ No    ☐ Maybe/Somewhat

9. Other ways to take care of brain health?

_____

   ☐ Yes    ☐ No    ☐ Maybe/Somewhat

10. Other ways to take care of brain health?

_____

   ☐ Yes    ☐ No    ☐ Maybe/Somewhat

**Notes:**

# Am I Having Memory Problems

## A 10-Week Journal – Week 10

Week: ☐ 1   ☐ 2   ☐ 3   ☐ 4   ☐ 5   ☐ 6   ☐ 7   ☐ 8   ☐ 9   ☐ 10

Today's date is: _____

☐ Monday  ☐ Tuesday  ☐ Wednesday  ☐ Thursday  ☐ Friday

☐ Saturday  ☐ Sunday

Big and small activities of the week or day:

_____

## Keeping Track of What I Am Forgetting

**My Memory issues/Forgetfulness this week:**

Did I forget something or have concerns about my memory today?

☐ Yes          ☐ No          ☐ Maybe

**This week, did I forget or have trouble with:** *(check if you had problems)*

**Forgetfulness:**

☐ Names      ☐ Keys      ☐ Wallet/bag/money      ☐ Cell phone

☐ What I wanted to say   ☐ Something else important_____

**Location:**

☐ Forgot day of the week   ☐ Forgot where I was

---

Am I Having Memory Problems and Am I Taking Care of My Brain Health: A 10 Week Journal from *Dear Dad, Can We Talk About Your Memory* by Tara Rose, PhD, © 2019. Permission to photocopy is granted with purchase of book, see copyright page.

**Felt confused**:

☐ What was I about to do   ☐ How to do something I normally do

**Lost:**

☐ Couldn't remember how to get somewhere

**Basics**:

☐ Problem getting dressed         ☐ How to cook or get a meal

☐ How to pay a bill

**What did I have problems with?**

_____

☐ I had memory problems but I don't remember what they were

**Notes**

# Am I Taking Care of my Brain Health?

## A 10-Week Journal – Week 10

Week: ☐ 1  ☐ 2  ☐ 3  ☐ 4  ☐ 5  ☐ 6  ☐ 7  ☐ 8  ☐ 9  ☐ 10

Today's date is: _____

☐ Monday  ☐ Tuesday  ☐ Wednesday  ☐ Thursday  ☐ Friday
☐ Saturday  ☐ Sunday

Big and small activities of the week or day:

_____

## Keeping Track of Healthy Brain Health

**Brain Health:  ☐ Today I:  ☐ This week I:**

1. Drank enough water and made sure I was hydrated?

  ☐ Yes          ☐ No          ☐ Maybe/Somewhat

2. Ate healthy?

  ☐ Yes          ☐ No          ☐ Maybe/Somewhat

3. Took my medication and/or vitamins for the day?

  ☐ Yes          ☐ No          ☐ Maybe/Somewhat

4. Had enough / good sleep last night?

  ☐ Yes          ☐ No          ☐ Maybe/Somewhat

5. Had stress?

    ☐ Yes      ☐ No      ☐ Maybe/Somewhat

    Managed the stress well?

    ☐ Yes      ☐ No      ☐ Maybe/Somewhat

6. Did body exercise (walk, aerobics, etc.)?

    ☐ Yes      ☐ No      ☐ Maybe/Somewhat

7. Had some kind of brain exercise?

    ☐ Yes      ☐ No      ☐ Maybe/Somewhat

8. Had social time / time with family or friends?

    ☐ Yes      ☐ No      ☐ Maybe/Somewhat

9. Other ways to take care of brain health?

_____

    ☐ Yes      ☐ No      ☐ Maybe/Somewhat

10. Other ways to take care of brain health?

_____

    ☐ Yes      ☐ No      ☐ Maybe/Somewhat

**Notes:**

## Spanish Translation – Traducción en español

### Querido Papá, Querías Saber Más Acerca de las Preocupaciones que Tienes Sobre tu Memoria

#### Una Guía sobre Qué Hacer y Un diario de Salud

**Tara Rose, PhD**

**Monica Miranda Schaeubinger, MD, MSPH**

*Sobre la traducción: La Dra. Mónica Miranda Schaeubinger es médica epidemióloga, nacida en la Ciudad de México. Ella tiene un gran interés por la promoción de la salud y la prevención de enfermedades. Actualmente, su trabajo de investigación se enfoca en la salud materna e infantil. Ella vive actualmente en Filadelfia, Estados Unidos.*

Dear Dad, Can We Talk About Your Memory?
Wisdom on Brain Health

**Tara Rose, PhD**
**Monica Miranda Schaeubinger, MD, MSPH**

About Translation: Dr. Mónica Miranda Schaeubinger is a physician epidemiologist. She is originally from Mexico City, and has great interest in health promotion and disease prevention. Her current research focuses on maternal and child health. She lives in Philadelphia, USA.

DEAR DAD, CAN WE TALK ABOUT YOUR MEMORY?

# Introducción

Esta es una carta del tipo "Querido Papá".

Se la escribí a mi papá después de visitarlo, ya que él tenía algunos problemas con su memoria. Los problemas no eran muy serios, pero, aun así, él se percató de ellos, y se empezó a preocupar. Esta es una carta de amor de una hija a su padre, algo informal pero que incluye información médica detallada que es algo típico en tal correspondencia. Mi padre y yo éramos profesionales trabajando en hospitales a lo largo de nuestras carreras, y este era mi campo de expertica: educación sobre Demencia y Alzheimer; es por ello que quise ayudarlo a conocer más sobre lo último en investigaciones sobre estos padecimientos.

SI bien escribí esta carta para mi papá, nunca se la entregué – él falleció un par de meses después (nada relacionado a sus problemas con la memoria). Cuando compartí esta carta y las hojas de trabajo "¿Estoy teniendo problemas de memoria" y "¿Estoy cuidando la salud de mi cerebro?" por primera vez, sentí que de alguna manera estaba honrando a mi padre. Han pasado tres años y he continuado actualizado la información. A la vez, he logrado mantener mi narrativa original como hija hablando con mi padre.

Quisiera darle una advertencia al lector: esta carta es muy técnica, por lo que sería recomendable saber algo sobre mi padre y yo: mi papá era un farmacéutico retirado y administrador principal de un hospital, por lo que la carta está escrita, a grandes rasgos, por alguien que tiene conocimientos avanzados en temas médicos. Soy psicóloga clínica especializada en gerontología y trabajo en uno de los centros de "The Alzheimer's Disease Research Center (ADRC)" (Centro de Investigación del Alzheimer) en los Estados Unidos. Por lo tanto, tengo experiencia en el área; está en mi campo el educar a otros, y por eso quise pasarle información a él. Y ahora, a usted. Si hay algo que no entienda, simplemente brínqueselo por ahora, y podría consultarlo después con su médico o proveedor de salud.

Es importante recalcar que esto es un libro. Por favor, compártaselo a sus padres si lo ve apropiado. También puede compartirlo con algún primo, prima tío, tía amigos o su pareja.

Lo invito a utilizar la información mostrada en esta carta; sin embargo, recuerde que es muy importante acudir a un doctor si tiene problemas de memoria. Lleve esta carta y su diario (ya completo) con su médico. No tome esta carta ni sus contenidos como una consulta médica. Sin embargo, léalo con cuidado y cuide de si mismo.

Los problemas de memoria serios no forman parte de un envejecimiento normal. Existen muchas maneras de revertir los síntomas de memoria, protegerse de padecer demencia y retrasar el desarrollo de problemas serios de memoria si es que usted tiene algún padecimiento.

Cuídese y que se encuentre bien,

Tara Rose

## Preguntas que tienes sobre tus recientes problemas de memoria

Querido Papá,

Me dijiste que estabas teniendo problemas de memoria y que tenías algunas preguntas. Pensé que sería más fácil darte algún consejo si lo escribo en una carta. Sabes que estoy en el campo de investigación del Alzheimer y de trastornos de la memoria, por lo que tengo muchos consejos para darte. Y siendo tu hija, pienso que son buenos consejos. Por eso, sólo escúchame y ten en cuenta que lo que te digo viene desde el fondo de mi corazón, pero al mismo tiempo tiene un enfoque académico, que, si bien tiene algunas limitaciones, 30 años de investigación sobre la enfermedad del Alzheimer parece un buen punto para empezar.

Permíteme comenzar con la etiqueta de "problemas de memoria". Me preguntaste qué es lo que el doctor haría si él determinara que tu nivel de padecimiento de memoria es un problema. Es posible que diría que tienes "deterioro cognitivo leve" (DCL). Sé que muchas personas se preocupan con desarrollar la enfermedad del Alzheimer o padecer demencia al envejecer. Sin embargo, esta carta no se trata sobre la enfermedad de Alzheimer o de demencia, y no saltemos a conclusiones simplemente porque estás teniendo algunos problemas de memoria. En vez de eso, quería hablarte sobre lo que significa realmente tener "deterioro cognitivo leve" (DCL) o problemas de memoria. Te diré sobre lo que investigadores y expertos en el área médica están diciendo sobre el DCL de tal manera de que te puedas informar sobre la investigación más reciente, tener la información, y quizás te brinde tranquilidad el informa sobre los hechos que te ayudarán a seguir adelante.

Permíteme empezar con una visión general de lo que se sabe actualmente sobre los problemas leves de memoria.

El deterioro cognitivo leve (DCL) significa que estás sufriendo cambios importantes en tu memoria y en tu raciocinio, que es lo que me has contado sobre tu caso; no obstante, estos cambios no son lo suficientemente severos ni serios como para requerir asistencia en tus actividades cotidianas. A veces, este nivel de problemas de memoria es también llamado "trastorno neurocognitivo leve" (mNCD en inglés) y es definido como una decremento notorio en el funcionamiento cognitivo que sobrepasa los cambios normales del envejecimiento. Recuerda: ¡Esto no es demencia ni Alzheimer!

Antes de continuar, tengo que contarte sobre qué es el Alzheimer y qué es la demencia, para que sepas porque estamos diciendo que tú no tienes ninguna de estas enfermedades, que son más serias.

La demencia (antiguamente conocido como demencia senil), significa que tienes problemas significativamente serios de memoria. La demencia es un conjunto de síntomas o problemas que alguien experimenta. Específicamente, es la pérdida de la capacidad de pensar, recordar y razonar (funcionamiento cognitivo), y de realizar las actividades diarias (habilidades conductuales) a tal punto de que interfiere con el día a día de una persona. Hay un rango de severidad de demencia que va desde el estado más leve, cuando comienza a afectar seriamente las funciones de las actividades cotidianas de una persona, hasta el estado más serio, en el cual una persona depende completamente de los demás para realizar sus actividades diarias.

El Alzheimer es una de las principales causas de la demencia, pero la única causa. El Alzheimer está caracterizado por las "placas y ovillos" que se pueden ver en el cerebro. Las placas son la acumulación de proteínas en algunas áreas del cerebro, y los ovillos se observan cuando la estructura de las neuronas sufre cambios que eventualmente llevan a la muerte de la neurona. De esta manera, el diagnóstico de demencia significa que hay síntomas de una perdida seria de la memoria y el

Alzheimer es una de sus posibles causas. Hay múltiples enfermedades que puedan causar demencia.

**El diagnóstico de la demencia o el Alzheimer es una situación más seria que el DCL (deterioro cognitivo leve).**

Estoy tratando de ser reconfortante. No estoy segura de qué tan bien lo estoy haciendo ... Aquí hay una imagen:

**Niveles de Problemas de Memoria:**

**• Primero, problemas de memoria REGULARES a medida que envejecemos**

**• Segundo, problemas de memoria MÁS GRANDES llamados deterioro cognitivo leve (DCL)**

**• Tercero, problemas de memoria GRAVES llamados demencia o enfermedad de Alzheimer.**

Es todo.

<u>**Diagnóstico, Tratamiento y Pronóstico**</u>

Permíteme decirte lo que nosotros (clínicos e investigadores) sabemos sobre el diagnóstico, tratamiento y pronóstico a largo plazo del tipo de problemas de memoria que podrías tener, llamado deterioro cognitivo leve (DCL).

En general, podemos decir que del 10% al 20% de las personas de 65 años o más tienen DCL o mNCD. Sabemos que el riesgo de desarrollar estos problemas aumenta con la edad, y que los hombres parecen presentar mayor riesgo que las mujeres.

Por lo tanto, a pesar de que las personas con DCL tienen un mayor riesgo de desarrollar demencia en comparación con cualquier persona en los Estados Unidos, existe un rango bastante amplio en las estimaciones de riesgo (<5% al 20% en tasas de conversión anual), según el grupo de personas o población estudiada. Una persona con diagnóstico de DCL, cada año tiene una probabilidad de recibir un diagnóstico de demencia que varía desde menos del 5% al 20%. Esto significa que algunas personas mejoran, otras permanecen igual y es cierto que la memoria de algunas personas empeora. Como tu hija, obviamente deseo que tu memoria mejore. Hay muchas cosas que pueden estar afectando tu memoria, así que tomemos medidas para que tu memoria "habitual" se recupere.

Hay varias razones por las cuales las personas mayores pueden tener DCL o un riesgo incrementado de desarrollar problemas de memoria, pensamiento y raciocinio, que incluyen sentirse triste o deprimido (depresión), tomar múltiples medicamentos que interactúan entre sí (polifarmacia) y problemas con el corazón y el flujo sanguíneo en el cuerpo (factores de riesgo cardiovascular no controlados).

Estos factores deben ser examinados y tomados en consideración por tu médico o proveedor de atención primaria.

Entonces, papá, si no te ocupas de la situación ahora que tus problemas de memoria son reversibles, existe la posibilidad de que más adelante se conviertan en daños permanentes - ¡así que cuídate y consulta a tu médico de inmediato!

Como puedes ver, el gran mensaje de esta carta es: ¡Ve a ver a tu médico! Así como que te cuides a ti mismo, a tu bienestar y a tu salud. Ahora, me gustaría indicarte cómo puedes comenzar a cuidar de tu salud y tu memoria y qué te platicaré qué debes tener en cuenta cuando visites a tu médico.

## ¿QUÉ PUEDE AYUDAR AHORA? ¡CUÍDATE!

¿Qué es lo mejor que puedes hacer para disminuir el riesgo de desarrollar más problemas de memoria?

Lo primero es lo primero, cuida de tu cuerpo y de tu cerebro. Como sabrás, están conectados. Cuidar de nosotros mismos puede crear cambios físicos positivos en el cerebro. Es realmente sorprendente y la investigación tiene solo unos pocos años. Hay mucha investigación nueva sobre cómo adquiriendo ciertos hábitos saludables específicos (de los ensayos clínicos), el cerebro puede cambiar y mejorar su funcionamiento. De hecho, se puede ver y medir los cambios en el cerebro escaneando los cerebros de las personas antes de comenzar el estudio de investigación, durante la intervención con la nueva actividad / hábito y finalmente, cuando se completa el estudio. Los investigadores ahora pueden ver qué áreas importantes del cerebro efectivamente crecen o se vuelven más saludables. Es como si ejercitaras y levantaras pesas. Tú has visto cómo tus músculos de los brazos o las piernas crecen y se vuelven más fuertes con ejercicio. Lo mismo pasa en tu cerebro. La diferencia es que no podemos mirar dentro del cerebro para ver los cambios, a menos de que usemos imágenes que cuestan miles de dólares. Debido a que puede llevar tiempo para que se sienta el cambio derivado de la mejoría de nuestras neuronas, puede ser fácil rendirse. Pero, cuando nos damos cuenta de que nuestra memoria mejora con el tiempo, es fácil entender que vale la pena establecer nuevos hábitos y mantenerlos.

No voy a escribir mucho sobre cada tema en la siguiente lista porque existen muchos libros sobre esos temas. Sólo quiero que sepas qué áreas para mantenerte saludable existen que cuentan con el respaldo de estudios de investigación. Sé que se necesita mucho esfuerzo para cambiar estas cosas y agregar nuevas actividades a nuestras vidas. También hay áreas en las que yo misma podría trabajar, así que quizás podamos hacer algunas juntos, aunque no estemos en la misma ciudad.

**1) Comer sano y bebe suficiente agua.** Come alimentos que sean buenos para tu corazón. Puedes buscar alimentos "saludables para el corazón" en Internet, e incluyen frutas y verduras, granos integrales, nueces, carnes magras y pescado. Se habla mucho sobre la "dieta mediterránea". Hay algunos estudios que han encontrado que vitaminas y nutrientes específicos pueden mejorar la salud, por lo que te iré contando más a medida que salga la investigación. En este momento, puedo decir que obtener suficiente Omega-3 es muy importante y obtenerlo del pescado parece ser la mejor fuente, por ejemplo, en pescado graso como el salmón, la caballa y las sardinas. No hay aún ninguna investigación que yo conozca sobre los alimentos orgánicos versus no orgánicos, pero dado que tienes algunos problemas de memoria, creo que deberías gastar un poco más en alimentos orgánicos (alimentos cultivados sin pesticidas ni aditivos) tanto como te sea posible. Tenemos la suerte de poder pagar ese gasto adicional, y dado que tu cerebro está pidiendo ayuda, por favor, no agregues productos químicos que puedan dañar el cuerpo.

También quiero mencionar otra área que no tiene suficiente investigación, la cual consiste en tomar una buena multi-vitamina y suplementos (si su proveedor los recomienda). Por favor tómalos. Parece que incluso si no tenemos la investigación en este momento, un cuerpo necesita todas las ventajas que pueda obtener para ayudar a la memoria.

Beber suficiente agua y mantenerse hidratado es importante, ya que la deshidratación realmente puede causar problemas de memoria.

**2) Ejercicio.** Asumiendo que tu médico diga que está bien hacer ejercicio, un plan de ejercicio que incluya actividades que aumenten tu ritmo cardíaco y también actividades consideradas como entrenamiento de fuerza (pesas y ejercicios de resistencia) sería lo mejor.

El ejercicio es el área más sorprendente para obtener beneficios, y existe investigación impresionante sobre este tema que incluye imágenes cerebrales que muestran cómo no solo cambia la estructura de tu corazón y músculos. sino que también cambia la estructura de tu cerebro con el ejercicio,

**3) Dormir lo suficiente**. Si no sueles poder dormir lo suficiente, lee sobre todas las formas de dormir mejor o consúltalo con tu proveedor de atención médica. Me encanta la analogía que describe el sueño como cuando llega el camión de basura y recoge toda la basura de tu cerebro que no debería estar allí. No canceles el servicio de recolección de basura al no dormir lo suficiente. Incluso, hay estudios de investigación que demuestran lo mencionado.

**4) Pasar tiempo con amigos y familiares**. Socializa y habla con los demás. Ten conversaciones con otras personas. Hay estudios que muestran que la actividad social está relacionada a tasas más bajas de disminución de la memoria, lo que significa que tu memoria permanece mejor por más tiempo. Los investigadores han demostrado que aquellas personas que tienen mayor contacto con otras rinden mejor en pruebas de memoria.

**5) Participar en la reducción de riesgos.** La reducción del riesgo significa dejar de hacer cosas que sabemos que son malas para nuestro cuerpo y que no son buenas para nuestro corazón. Fumar es un buen ejemplo. Sabemos que esto es malo para nuestra salud en general, y, de hecho, también puede afectar nuestro cerebro.

Un corazón sano es muy importante para nuestro cerebro, lo cual tiene sentido. Necesitamos que la sangre llegue del corazón al cerebro, por lo que necesitamos un corazón sano. Y la sangre también transporta la glucosa o el azúcar en la sangre al cerebro - es la energía para el cerebro. Por lo tanto, si alguien tiene un nivel inadecuado de azúcar en la sangre, ya sea demasiado alto o demasiado bajo, este puede causar problemas en la conductividad funcional en el cerebro y causar problemas de memoria.

    A.  **Dejar de fumar**. Si estás fumando de nuevo, intenta dejarlo. Además, procura mantenerte alejado de personas que estén

73

fumando, porque el humo de segunda mano también es perjudicial.

**B. Diabetes.** ¿Te han revisado el azúcar en la sangre? Ahora sabemos que la diabetes, e incluso la prediabetes (cuando los niveles de azúcar en la sangre están altos pero no lo suficientemente altos como para clasificarse como diabetes) está relacionada con la demencia. Reduce también el consumo de azúcar procesado, por favor.

**C. Presión arterial alta o hipertensión**. Controlar tu presión arterial es realmente importante. Piénsalo: tener mayor presión en las arterias que van al cerebro de lo que deberías no suena como algo bueno para nosotros.

**D. Depresión y ansiedad.** Algunos estudios de investigación muestran que las personas que sufren de depresión y ansiedad tienen más probabilidades de tener problemas de memoria. No sabemos con certeza por qué, pero esto significa que es beneficioso tratar esos sentimientos y recibir ayuda. Hay muchos tratamientos para estos padecimientos si estás experimentando alguno de ellos ahora.

**E. Inflamación.** La inflamación en el cuerpo no es buena para nosotros. La inflamación de la parte del cuerpo donde la sangre se filtra para formar el líquido cefalorraquídeo (llamada barrera hematoencefálica) es especialmente malo. Si la barrera hematoencefálica, esa pequeña "puerta" donde el líquido cefalorraquídeo ingresa al cerebro, tiene inflamación, entonces este se puede alterar y eso significa que otras cosas pueden ingresar al cerebro y causar estragos en del cerebro. Por ello, es importante que cuides tu cuerpo, incluso ir al dentista para evitar la enfermedad de las encías (que es un tipo de inflamación en el cuerpo).

**6. Ejercitar tu cerebro.** Es cierto que al igual que nuestro cuerpo necesita ejercicio, nuestro cerebro también. Dale a tu mente actividades mentalmente desafiantes. Puede ser lo que quieras. Jugar juegos, hacer rompecabezas, leer, aprender cosas nuevas, tener un pasatiempo. También podría ser formar parte de un voluntariado para ayudar a otros, especialmente con la jubilación.

**7. Reducir el estrés.** El estrés crónico puede dañar al cerebro, lo que dificulta el aprendizaje y causa problemas de memoria. Se ha demostrado que la meditación, el yoga y otras actividades de mente y cuerpo alivian diferentes problemas. La meditación y el yoga pueden incluso cambiar la estructura de nuestro cerebro y reducir la inflamación en el cerebro en las áreas de la memoria.

**8. Música**. A ti te encanta la música, así que escucha tus canciones favoritas o canta. Creo que te hará más feliz. Hay nuevos estudios que muestran cómo la música estimula diferentes partes del cerebro.

**9. Ama y sé agradecido.** Ora y se agradecido. Tú me lo enseñaste en mi vida, así que ¿puedo decírtelo yo ahora? Toma asiento y respira, ve con Dios, como sea que tu lo hagas. No estoy segura sobre lo que indica la investigación sobre este último punto, pero no puedo imaginar un mejor consejo.

Hay muchas ideas para la salud del cerebro. Elige lo que funciona para ti ahora mismo.

### Ver a un médico o proveedor de atención

Bien, ahora hablemos acerca de ir al médico o al proveedor de atención médica para revisar tus problemas de memoria. Esto es muy importante. Voy a ser técnico en esta sección, pero dado que ambos hemos trabajado en hospitales, creo que preferiría incluir más detalles que puedan ser útiles. Si no estás seguro sobre algunos de mis puntos, entonces pregúntale a tu médico para que te lo explique.

**Para la cita**

Asegúrate de **traer a alguien** contigo a la cita con el médico.

Este es un consejo importante. Ayudaría si pudieras llevar a alguien cercano a ti, que te conozca bien (como mamá), que pueda confirmar tus problemas de memoria y transmitir el mensaje de que quieres que el médico tome en serio tus preocupaciones. Mamá (o quien sea que traigas) también puede tomar notas, de tal manera que tú solo te tengas que preocupar en escuchar al doctor.

**¿Qué debe verificar el médico si tienes problemas de memoria o DCL?**

El médico debe saber sobre los siguientes aspectos de tu vida: (Sería bueno que escribas algunas notas y una lista antes de ir a la cita).

1. Cambios en la memoria / función cognitiva (cuando empezó, cómo ha cambiado, ejemplos de problemas de memoria).

2. Cambios en la capacidad para realizar actividades cotidianas. Esto incluye actividades de la vida diaria, o cómo llevas tu día y las dificultades que puedas enfrentar, incluyendo el manejo de las finanzas y la administración del dinero.

3. ¿Estás comiendo bien y cuánto estas bebiendo? Sí, ¡tanto agua como alcohol! Recuerda que estar deshidratado (no beber suficiente agua) puede causar problemas de memoria.

4. Recetas médicas y medicamentos disponibles a la venta sin receta médica. Esto incluye vitaminas y suplementos nutricionales.

5. Síntomas que pueden estar relacionados al cerebro, tales como: audición, visión, habla, problemas para dormir, caminar, entumecimiento u hormigueo en cualquier parte del cuerpo.

6. Síntomas relacionados con la salud del corazón - significa que el cerebro obtenga, de manera correcta, suficiente flujo de sangre del corazón hacia el cerebro y luego envíe la cantidad correcta de azúcar / glucosa en la sangre y oxígeno hacia el cerebro. Mencioné esto anteriormente, por lo tanto, si tienes algún padecimiento como presión arterial alta, prediabetes o diabetes, o algún problema cardíaco, incluidos latidos cardíacos irregulares, prepárate para discutirlos con el médico.

7. Problemas de salud mental o bienestar, como depresión, ansiedad, cambios en la personalidad o la conducta que pueden causar problemas de memoria.

8. Antecedentes familiares. El médico también querrá saber sobre nuestra historia familiar. Hasta donde sé, somos afortunados, ya que no tenemos antecedentes familiares de deterioro en la memoria o demencia. Pero, Papá, si sabes algo de la familia, díselo al médico.

**El médico o proveedor de salud querrá realizar un examen físico y también te hará un examen neurológico.** Quiero que el médico tenga la oportunidad de hacerte preguntas y realizarte un examen físico para ver qué está pasando.

### Pruebas de Sangre de Laboratorio

Solicita trabajos de laboratorio o pruebas de laboratorio que sean de rutina para alguien de tu edad, ya que tus problemas de memoria podrían deberse por alguna condición, o bien deficiencia de vitaminas o de minerales, lo cual podría afectar tu memoria.

Estas son las pruebas que se que deberías solicitar que te realicen, al menos si tienes seguro médico: análisis de sangre que incluya un panel metabólico completo, necesita incluir: biometría hemática, electrolitos, glucosa, calcio, función tiroidea, hierro, vitamina B12 y folato. Pero tu médico podría querer hacer más pruebas de otros aspectos de tu sangre.

La razón por la que quisieras que todas estas pruebas se realicen en tu sangre es para identificar maneras posiblemente reversibles de DCL, incluyendo infección, problemas renales, muy poco o demasiado magnesio, muy poco o demasiado calcio, problemas de nivel de alto glucosa / azúcar en la sangre (hiperglucemia), problemas de tiroides y problemas de vitaminas o nutrientes (deficiencia de vitamina B12, hierro o folato). No será una sorpresa descubrir que tienes alguno de estos de la lista dada la dieta estadounidense (mala broma para ti).

Pruebas de laboratorio adicionales pueden verificar la función renal y la función hepática. Además, la enfermedad de Lyme, la sífilis y el VIH pueden revelar causas más raras del deterioro cognitivo. Pero solo para que sepas, es posible que el médico no comience con estas pruebas o que nunca realice pruebas de enfermedades de transmisión sexual a menos que digas algo (aquí espero que te rías).

También hay pruebas de laboratorio para la apnea del sueño, cuando y si roncas o tienes problemas para respirar regularmente por la noche, lo que puede afectar tu capacidad de concentración y tu memoria durante el día.

**Revisión Profesional de Medicamentos: ¿Por qué?**

Lo que tú quieres es una revisión profesional de medicamentos. Lo sabes debido a que eres farmacéutico y es particularmente importante para las personas con problemas de memoria. Ciertas clases y combinaciones de medicamentos pueden

contribuir a los problemas de memoria y deterioro cognitivo, por lo que se deben revisar todas las recetas actuales, medicamentos de venta sin receta médica y vitaminas.

Probablemente no necesitas saber esto ahora, pero las clases de medicamentos que tienen más probabilidades de contribuir al deterioro cognitivo incluyen los anticolinérgicos, opiáceos, benzodiazepinas y fármacos hipnóticos no benzodiazepínicos (por ejemplo, Zolpidem), digoxina, antihistamínicos, antidepresivos tricíclicos, relajantes del musculares y antiepilépticos. Se ha demostrado que la terapia hormonal (estrógeno solo o estrógeno más progestágenos) para la menopausia aumenta el riesgo para el resultado combinado de DCL o demencia (no es que realmente se aplique a ti, pero te podría resultar interesante). Además, los hipotensivos utilizados para tratar la hipertensión (presión arterial alta) y medicamentos para ;ps problemas de azúcar en la sangre, incluyendo la hipoglucemia, la hiperglucemia, la prediabetes (resultados elevados de azúcar en la sangre) y la diabetes, también pueden contribuir a problemas cognitivos.

## Prueba Cognitiva o de Memoria

Queremos que alguien haga pruebas de memoria o cognitivas contigo. El profesional de la salud también realizará pruebas cognitivas o de memoria muy básicas, que demoran entre 10 a 20 minutos. Hay varias pruebas diferentes que el médico podría realizar, por ejemplo una prueba llamada Evaluación Cognitiva Montreal (MoCA en inglés), el Instrumento de Evaluación Mini-Cognitiva (Mini-Cog), o mi favorito, la prueba de 3MS (Estado Mini Mental Modificado). Si el médico quiere hacer más pruebas, simplemente alégrate de que estas obteniendo una mejor y más completa evaluación. Será útil tener esos resultados. Y si el médico vuelve a hablar contigo dentro de seis meses o un año, podrás ver cómo cambió tu memoria o si se mantuvo igual. Tu primera prueba de memoria se llama de base y, de nuevo, es muy útil hacerla.

## Solicita escaneos cerebrales: Imágenes de tu Cerebro

La tecnología es increíble ahora, y si parece que sufres de problemas de memoria, entonces el médico puede ordenar algunos escaneos cerebrales - o imágenes de tu cerebro. Por favor accede a esto. No duele, y solo tienes que quedarte quieto durante 30 a 45 minutos en una máquina, y ellos tomarán imágenes de tu cerebro.

Hay un par de tipos de pruebas diferentes que crean imágenes de tu cerebro. Una resonancia magnética (RM) o tomografía computarizada (también llamada TAC por tomografía axial computarizada) ambas son pruebas apropiadas. Por lo general, el médico solo ordena uno o más.

¿Por qué hacen este tipo de escaneos cerebrales? Para observar que no hay masa (tumor), hemorragia o infección. Como todos nuestros cerebros se reducen, los médicos también observan el "volumen cerebral" para verificar que la pérdida o la reducción en volumen sea acorde a tu edad, y no más que eso. También buscan otros tipos de cambios cerebrales o estructurales para asegurarse de que no haya nada inusual.

Es bueno tener estas y otras pruebas como una "base", tal cual como mencioné anteriormente, y si todavía tiene problemas de memoria en un año o dos y no se resuelven por sí solos, el médico puede realizar otro escaneo y luego puede comparar los resultados.

Otra buena razón para realizarte el escaneo **es que, si has tenido un accidente cerebrovascular (infarto cerebral o derrame cerebral). un impulso silencioso (es decir, uno que uno no percibe) o un ataque isquémico transitorio (AIT),** podrías ya sea experimentar pérdida de memoria, pero podrías recuperar algo o la mayoría del funcionamiento y memoria anteriores. Muchas veces estos derrames cerebrales se pueden ver en la tecnología de imágenes cerebrales y eso es importante porque querrás ver a un cardiólogo o neurólogo para reducir o dejar de tener estos problemas de salud - ¡y asegurarte de no volver a tener uno!

**¿Qué descubrimos de la evaluación y los resultados de las pruebas?**

Si alguno de los resultados o factores es significativo, el médico intentará tratar esos síntomas para ver si tu memoria mejora. El médico también querrá discutir lo que se encontró con respecto al diagnóstico de DCL contigo y otros miembros de la familia (o con quien vayas a la cita).

De cualquier manera, el médico querrá volver a verte en seis meses. Por lo tanto, es importante arreglar una cita de seguimiento aproximadamente cada seis meses para que el médico pueda observar los cambios (incluidas las mejoras) en la memoria / funciones cognitivas y también en las necesidades que tengas.

## Referencia médica, por favor, si es necesaria

Si tienes algún problema grave con la memoria, quiero que el médico de atención primaria / profesional de la salud te remita a un especialista, ya que los expertos son importantes y saben qué analizar y qué cosas pueden ayudarte. Esta persona suele ser un neurólogo o especialista en geriatría (alguien que trabaja con adultos mayores).

## Diagnóstico de deterioro cognitivo leve

## ¿Cuál es la información necesaria o los criterios para diagnosticar DCL?

Aquí está la información que el médico usa para diagnosticar el deterioro cognitivo leve (DCL), pero ten en cuenta que los criterios pueden cambiar:

1. Problema con respecto a un cambio en las habilidades de pensamiento (cognición) de la persona, de alguien que conoce a la persona o de un clínico que la ha observado.

2. "Evidencia objetiva" de discapacidad (ver las pruebas anteriores) en una o más áreas cognitivas, incluyendo la memoria, la función ejecutiva, la atención, el lenguaje o las habilidades visuales y espaciales.

3. Preservación de la independencia en las habilidades funcionales (aunque una persona puede ser menos eficiente y cometer más errores al realizar actividades de la vida diaria y actividades instrumentales de la vida cotidiana a comparación de antes).

4. Falta de evidencia de un impedimento significativo en el funcionamiento social u ocupacional (es decir, no tener demencia).

Espero que puedas ver que esta lista muestra algunos problemas, pero no problemas severos, que es lo que se denomina deterioro cognitivo leve hoy en día.

Eso es todo con respecto a lo que pueden hacer los proveedores de atención primaria o los médicos para ayudarte. Ahora quiero hablarte acerca de otras cosas que puedes hacer una vez que salgas del consultorio del médico para ayudar potencialmente a su memoria.

**Reserva una cita con tu médico de atención primaria / médico general, y si lo deseas, usa el diario de 10 semanas y las hojas de trabajo que incluyo a continuación y llévalas al médico.** Puedes completar el diario y las hojas de trabajo por ti mismo, pero a menudo es mejor que lo hagan otras personas cercanas a ti. Tal vez mamá pueda llenarlo por ti, o podríamos hacerlo por teléfono. Avísame.

**Espero que encuentres esto de utilidad. Me doy cuenta de que esta es una carta muy larga, pero quería que tuvieras la información ya que este es mi campo. Estoy cerca, solo llámame.**

**Te amo, papá. Estás en mis oraciones, y ojalá Dios te dé salud, bienestar y paz.**

**Con amor, mucho amor,**

**Tara Rose**

# ¿Estoy Teniendo Problemas de Memoria o Esto es Normal?

## Hoja de Trabajo

Completa esto antes de ir al consultorio de tu proveedor de atención médica y tráelo contigo a su cita. Los médicos no tienen tanto tiempo, al menos no como en los "viejos tiempos", por lo que sería útil que completes esto antes de ir a la cita y que se lo muestres al médico si se empieza a terminar el tiempo de la consulta.

Tu nombre:

_____

Doctor/ Proveedor de Salud: _____

Fecha de la cita:

_____

Número de teléfono del Doctor/Proveedor de Salud:

_____

**Me preocupa mi memoria. He escrito algunas notas y he completado este formulario sobre mis problemas de memoria. ¿Quiere que lea mis notas? Puede hacer una copia si quiere.**

**MEMORIA: Estoy preocupado sobre estas cosas y quisiera saber si esto es normal o no:**

Me preocupa mi memoria cuando yo _____

_____

También me preocupa mi memoria cuando yo _____

_____

Otra preocupación de la memoria que tengo es_____

_____

¿HAY ALLGO QUE MEJORE O EMPEORE LOS PROBLEMAS DE MEMORIA? ¿LOS PROBLEMAS DE LA MEMORIA ESTAN PRESENTES TODO EL TIEMPO O SÓLO ALGUNAS VECES (Y CUANDO)?

    1._____

    2. _____

¿CÓMO AFECTAN ESTOS PROBLEMAS DE MEMORIA MI VIDA COTIDIANA?

    1. _____

    2. _____

**Medicamentos, otros problemas físicos**

Problemas de salud mental o bienestar:

☐ Ansioso o Ansiedad   ☐ Tristeza o Depresión

_____

Otros problemas en su vida (lista corta) (cambios o cosas/eventos que son estresante o difíciles de manejar):

_____

_____

Apuntes:

**Aquí hay algunas cosas que puede decirle a su médico / profesional de la salud en su cita:**

"¿Me podría realizar una prueba de memoria en esta cita o en otra cita? Escuché que solo toma de 10 a 15 minutos y me gustaría saber si hay algún problema ".

"Si parece que puede haber un problema o una posible pregunta sobre mi memoria, me gustaría que me hagan un análisis de sangre para asegurarme de que no tengo ninguna causa de problemas de memoria que sea reversible, como una deficiencia de vitaminas. Aquí hay una carta que mi hija escribió que enumera los tipos de análisis de sangre que podría necesitar ".

"¿Podría revisar los medicamentos que actualmente tomo para asegurarme de que no haya interacciones medicamentosas entre ellos?"

---

¿Estoy Teniendo Problemas de Memoria o Esto es Normal? Hoja de Trabajo. En *Dear Dad, Can We Talk About Your Memory* by Tara Rose, PhD, © 2019. Permission to photocopy is granted with purchase of book

DEAR DAD, CAN WE TALK ABOUT YOUR MEMORY?

# ¿Estoy Teniendo Problemas de Memoria?

## Un Diario de 10 Semanas

**Semana** ☐ 1  ☐ 2  ☐ 3  ☐ 4  ☐ 5  ☐ 6  ☐ 7  ☐ 8  ☐ 9  ☐ 10

**Hoy es:** _____

☐ 1  ☐ 2  ☐ 3  ☐ 4  ☐ 5  ☐ 6  ☐ 7  ☐ 8  ☐ 9  ☐ 10

☐ **Lunes**  ☐ **Martes**  ☐ **Miércoles**  ☐ **Jueves**  ☐ **Viernes**

☐ **Sábado**  ☐ **Domingo**    ☐ **Esta semana:**    ☐ **Hoy:**

**Actividades grandes y pequeñas del día o semana:**

_____

## Seguimiento de lo que olvido

**Mis problemas de memoria/olvido de hoy:**

¿Olvidaste algo o has tenido problemas con tu memoria el día de hoy?

☐ Si  ☐ No  ☐ Tal vez/Algo

**Hoy, ¿Tuve problemas u olvidé algo sobre: (marca con lo que tienes problemas)?**

**Olvido:**

☐ Nombres    ☐ Llaves    ☐ Billetera/maleta    ☐ Celular

☐ Lo que quería decir    ☐ Otra cosa importante

**Lugar y tiempo:**

☐ Olvide el día de la semana    ☐ Olvidé donde estaba

Am I Having Memory Problems and Am I Taking Care of My Brain Health: A 10 Week Journal, En *Dear Dad, Can We Talk About Your Memory* by Tara Rose, PhD, © 2019. Permission to photocopy is granted with purchase of book

**Me siento confundido**:

☐ Qué es lo que iba a hacer

☐ Cómo hacer algo que normalmente hago

**Ubicación:**

☐ No puedo recordar cómo llegar a algún lado

**Básicos**:

☐ Problemas al vestirme    ☐ Como pedir o cocinar mis comidas

☐ Cómo pagar una factura

**¿Con qué tuviste problemas?**

_____

☐ Tuve problemas de memoria, pero no recuerdo cuales eran.

Apuntes:

## ¿Estoy Cuidando la salud de mi cerebro?

## Un Diario de 10 Semanas

Semana ☐ 1  ☐ 2  ☐ 3  ☐ 4  ☐ 5  ☐ 6  ☐ 7  ☐ 8  ☐ 9  ☐ 10

Hoy es: _____

☐ 1  ☐ 2  ☐ 3  ☐ 4  ☐ 5  ☐ 6  ☐ 7  ☐ 8  ☐ 9  ☐ 10

☐ Lunes  ☐ Martes  ☐ Miércoles  ☐ Jueves  ☐ Viernes

☐ Sábado  ☐ Domingo        ☐ Esta semana:    ☐ Hoy:

**Actividades grandes y pequeñas del día o semana:**

_____

## Seguimiento de actividades para un cerebro sano

**Salud del cerebro:** ☐ Hoy yo:  ☐ Esta semana yo:

1. ¿Bebí suficiente agua y me aseguré de mantenerme hidratado?

   ☐ Si  ☐ No  ☐ Tal vez/Algo

2. ¿Comí saludablemente?

   ☐ Si  ☐ No  ☐ Tal vez/Algo

3. ¿Tome mis medicamentos y/o vitaminas del día?

   ☐ Si  ☐ No  ☐ Tal vez/Algo

4. ¿Descansé lo suficiente la noche anterior?

   ☐ Si  ☐ No  ☐ Tal vez/Algo

5. ¿Tuve estrés?

☐ Si   ☐ No   ☐ Tal vez/Algo

¿Controlé bien el estrés?

☐ Si   ☐ No   ☐ Tal vez/Algo

6. ¿Hice ejercicio físico (caminar, aeróbicos, etc.)?

☐ Si   ☐ No   ☐ Tal vez/Algo

7. ¿Practiqué algún tipo de ejercicio mental?

☐ Si   ☐ No   ☐ Tal vez/Algo

8. ¿Tuve tiempo para socializar/ estar con familia y amigos?

☐ Si   ☐ No   ☐ Tal vez/Algo

9. Otras formas de cuidar la salud del cerebro?

_____

☐ Si   ☐ No   ☐ Tal vez/Algo

10. Otras formas de cuidar la salud del cerebro?

_____

☐ Si   ☐ No   ☐ Tal vez/Algo

Apuntes:

_____

Am I Having Memory Problems and Am I Taking Care of My Brain Health: A 10 Week Journal,  En *Dear Dad, Can We Talk About Your Memory* by Tara Rose, PhD, © 2019. Permission to photocopy is granted with purchase of book

## Chinese (Simplified Chinese/Mandarin) – 简体中文翻译版

亲爱的爸爸，您曾想了解的关于您的记忆力问题的更多信息

记忆力问题应对指引及健康自检日志

塔拉·罗丝

童传风

特别感谢以下人员的翻译工作：

蒋同戈，余磊，张耕

童传风是武汉大学中南医院心血管内科的主任医师，副教授，硕士生导师。

---

Dear Dad, Can We Talk About Your Memory?

Wisdom on Brain Health

Tara Rose, PhD

Tong Chuanfeng, MD

Special thanks for help with translation to:

Tongge Jiang, MA, Lei Yu, MA, and Geng Zhang, MA

About Translation: Dr. Tong Chuanfeng is a physician Zhongnan Hospital of Wuhan University. She is the director of the Department of Cardiology at  Zhongnan Hospital of Wuhan University.

---

DEAR DAD, CAN WE TALK ABOUT YOUR MEMORY?

# 介绍

这封信是我写给亲爱的爸爸的。

当他出现了一些记忆上的问题时，我去看望了他。虽然父亲的问题并不是很严重，但他已经在自己身上发现了记忆力下降的现象，这令我们很担心。回来后，我便写下了这封女儿致父亲的"情书"。这封信并不是什么正式的医学函件，但也包含了一些医学细节和专业的医疗信息。我的父亲和我都是在医院工作的专业人士，因为我的专业领域是老年痴呆症和阿尔茨海默症的科普教育，所以我为父亲写下这封信，想让他了解医学上对记忆力有关疾病的最新研究。

虽然我为父亲写了这封信，但这封信最后并没有交给父亲——他在几个月后就去世了（是与他的记忆力无关的问题）。后来，当我开始分享这封信的内容、分享这封信里的"我有记忆上的问题吗？"和"我在很好地照料大脑的健康吗？"两份自检日志时，我想这也是对父亲的某种纪念。现在，已经三年过去了，我重新整理了这封信，同时保留了我作为女儿，对深爱的父亲想要说的话。

我想先提醒读者，这封信是非常专业的，所以读者可能需要先了解我父亲和我的一些情况：父亲是一名退休的药剂师，他生前做到了医院的高级管理人员的位置。所以这封信的某些内容，可能只有对医学有着较深的理解的人才能轻松读懂。而我在美国一所阿尔茨海默症研究中心（ADRC）工作，是专门研究老龄学的临床心理学家。我的工作是教育别人有关阿尔茨海默症的知识，这是我的专长，所以我原本只想将有关阿尔茨海默症的一些信息，通过这封信告诉父亲。现在我想将这些信息在这里告诉更多的人。在读这封信时，请读者先跳过遇到的不明白的地方，在有机会时咨询医生或专业的医疗从业人员。

我希望更多的人能看到这本小册子。如果可以的话，我想请读者阅读后再将它分享给你的父母，或者是你的爷爷、奶奶、朋友或其它需要的人。

欢迎读者用这封信中的内容来关注自己和身边的人的健康。但请记住，当发现任何阿尔茨海默症的疑似症状时候，最重要的应该是去看医生。你可以将这本小册子和记录好的自检日志交给医生。这本小册子并不是医疗建议，但也请你仔细阅读并照顾好自己。严重的记忆问题并不是人衰老过程中的正常现象，而现在医学上有很多方法可以逆转记忆力的衰退，让人们远离老年痴呆症。即便你已经确诊患有这种疾病，也有许多办法可以延缓记忆力的严重衰退。

祝安，

塔拉·罗丝

Tara Rose

## 有关您最近记忆力问题的一些信息

亲爱的爸爸

您说您的记忆出现了问题，对此也有一些疑问。我把一些有关的建议写在了这封信里，我想这对您来讲最直接。您知道我是从事有关阿尔茨海默症和记忆问题的研究工作的，所以我在这方面能给您很多建议。并且作为您的女儿，我想这封信中的建议对您来说会有帮助。所以当您看到这些建议的时候，应该能明白它们是来自女儿内心的声音。同时，由于这些建议比较专注于学术，它们可能也会有一些局限性；但是这些信息，对于了解近 30 年医学上对阿尔茨海默症的研究，可能是一个很好的起点。

我先从您说的"记忆力出现问题"来解答您的疑惑。您问我，如果医生认为您的记忆力有问题，医生会做些什么。很可能医生会说您有"轻度认知障碍（MCI）"。我知道很多老人都会担心，自己会随着年龄的增长而患上阿尔茨海默症或老年痴呆症。但是，这封信并不是要讲得了阿尔茨海默症或老年痴呆症之后要如何如何，我们不要因为您有一些记忆问题就匆忙下结论。相反，在这封信里我想和您谈的是，记忆问题或轻度认知障碍的真正含义。所以，我要告诉您的是医学领域和研究人员目前对轻度认知障碍的看法，从而帮助您了解到最新的医学研究进展和最新的资讯。另外，了解一些如何让您有所好转的方法，可能会让您的内心更加放松。

我先讲讲目前业内医学人员对轻度认知障碍的看法。

轻度认知障碍（MCI）是指一个人的记忆力和思维发生了明显的变化，这也是您告诉我，您在自己身上发现的症状。然而，这种变化还没有严重到让您在日常活动中需要频繁的帮助的程度。有时，这种程度的记忆力问题也被称为"轻度神经 认知障碍"（mNCD），其定义是：认知功能的显著下降，其程度超过了正常年龄增长而导致的变化。请您记住：这不并等同于老年痴呆症或阿尔茨海默症！

95

在我继续往下讲之前，我必须告诉您什么是老年痴呆症和阿尔茨海默症。这样您就会明白为什么我不认为您属于其中一种或同时有这两种严重的疾病。

老年痴呆症（英文称为"Dementia"，过去也被称"老年病"），指一个人的记忆出现了严重的问题，是一个人的身上正出现一系列的病症和健康问题。具体地说，这个人的思维、记忆、推理（认知功能）和日常行动（行为能力）的能力受到了损害，且严重程度足以干扰其正常的日常生活和活动。在老年痴呆症最轻微的阶段，它只是开始严重影响病人每天的日常功能……发展到最严重的阶段时，病人的日常基本活动和日常生活必须完全依赖他人的帮助。

阿尔茨海默症是造成老年痴呆的主要原因之一，但并不是唯一的原因。阿尔茨海默症的病理特征是：在病人的大脑组织中能发现"斑块和缠结"。斑块是在大脑的特定区域出现了特定蛋白质堆积；缠结则是在大脑的重要细胞死亡时形成并占据大脑的某些区域。因此，痴呆的诊断意味着有严重的记忆丧失症状，阿尔茨海默病是痴呆的可能原因之一。多种疾病也可以导致痴呆

**与轻度认知障碍（MCI）相比，老年痴呆症或阿尔茨海默症更为严重。**

父亲，我想努力让您安心，我也不确定我做的能有多好……下面是这些健康问题与疾病的程度汇总：

## 记忆问题的分层

• **第一；常见记忆问题**：随着年龄的增长，人的记忆力普遍会出现的问题。

• **第二；轻度认知障碍（MCI）**：严重一些的记忆问题。

• **第三；痴呆症或阿尔茨海默症**：更加严重的记忆问题。

**诊断、治疗、预后**

接下来让我告诉您我们（临床医生和研究人员）所知道的关于你们所说的轻度认知障碍（MCI）之类记忆障碍的是诊断、治疗和长期预后。

总的来说，我们可以说，在 65 岁及以上的老年人中，有 10% 到 20% 的人会患有 MCI 或 mNCD。我们知道，患这些疾病的风险随着年龄的增长而增加，而且男性似乎比女性面临更高的风险。因此，尽管与美国其他人群相比，MIC 患者换痴呆症的风险更大，但根据研究人群或族群的情况，风险估计范围相当大（从 <5% 到 20% 的年转化率）这是说，如果一个人被诊断为轻度认知障碍，那么每年他再被诊断为老年痴呆的几率会从低于 5% 到 20% 之间。所以，即使都有轻度认知障碍，有些人会变得更好，有些人能保持不变，而有些人的记忆问题确实会变得日益严峻。父亲，作为您的女儿，我当然希望您的记忆力能好起来。实际上，有许多方法可以改善您的记忆力，所以让我们行动起来，让您的记忆力回到"正常"。

有很多方面的原因，会导致老年人出现轻度认知障碍，或导致记忆、思维和其它问题的风险增加。这当中包括悲伤或抑郁（抑郁症）、多种药物相互作用（多重用药），以及心脏和身体的血液流动的问题（未控制的心血管危险因素）。这需要您的医生或基本的医疗服务人员进行检查与诊断。

所以，父亲，如果您在记忆还能恢复的阶段不好好照护自己，这种问题可能会给您带来永久性的伤害——所以请照顾好自己，马上去看医生！

我想您看到这里也明白了，这封信里最重要的信息是您要去看医生！请您照顾好自己、照顾好自己的幸福和健康——并且从现在就开始行动。下面，我想告诉您要如何照顾自己健康、保护自己的记忆力，以及看医生时您要记住什么。

**现在应该做些什么有益的事？照顾好自己的身体！**

现在做些什么对您最有帮助，并且能够降低您的记忆问题恶化的风险？

最重要的，要照顾好自己的身体和大脑。您也知道，身体与大脑是紧密相关的。照顾好身体实际上可以给大脑带来积极的生理变化。这真的很神奇，这方面的研究才进行了几年。现在有许多新的研究，是关于特定的健康习惯（在临床试验中）会如何改变大脑和改善大脑功能。在研究开始前，医学人员通过扫描受试者的大脑来观察、测量和记录大脑的变化；然后用新的活动、习惯进行干预治疗；等到干预结束后，再重新扫描受试者的大脑。通过与以前的数据的比较，医学人员发现大脑的重要区域实际上在生长或变得更健康了。这就好像是，进行身体锻炼和举重，我们会看到手臂或大腿的肌肉在生长和变得强壮一样，大脑也是如此。不同之处是，如果我们不花数千美元对大脑进行医学影像检查的话我们将无法看到大脑内部的变化。因为记忆能力需要时间来恢复，所以我们很容易放弃这些有益的活动与习惯。但是，如果能够把这些有益的活动和习惯坚持下去，随着时间的推移，当记忆能力好转时，我们就会明白当初的坚持是值得的。

在这封信里，我不会在每个话题下说太多，有很多关于这些话题的书可以详细地告诉我们要怎么做。我只是想让您知道，有哪些基本的方面可以帮助您保持健康并变得更健康，其中哪些是有科学研究依据的。我知道要做出改变、适应新的活动与习惯、在生活中加入新的东西，需要努力也需要坚持。有些方面我可以为您做，即使我们不在同一个城市，我们也可以一起做一些事情。

**1）吃得健康、多喝水**。多吃对心脏有益的食物。您可以在网上查找"有益心脏健康"的食物。水果、蔬菜、全谷物、坚果、瘦肉和鱼，这些都于人的身体健康有益。您可以关注一下公认健康的"地中海饮食"习惯。有些研究表明特定的维生素和营养剂可以改善人体健康，以后我将告诉您更多新的研究结果。而现在，摄入足够的 Omega-3 脂肪酸是很重要的，而从鱼类脂肪中提取的 Omega-3 脂肪酸似乎是最好的来源。所以鲑鱼（三文鱼）、鲭鱼和沙丁鱼等富含脂肪的鱼类都是不错的食物。据我所知，目前还没有任何关于有机食品和非有机食品对记忆力的影响的研究。但既然您有一点记忆力的问题，我认为您应该尽可能食用有机食品（不含杀虫剂或添加剂的食品）。我们都很幸运，经济宽裕能够负担得起额外的开销。现在考虑到您大脑的健康需要，请您不要吃含有可能伤害身体的化学物质的食品。

我还想说说另一个还没有足够研究的领域，那就是服用多种维生素和营养品的作用（您的健康服务方也做过这样的建议）。请服用它们，即使现在还没有相关的研究证据，但我们的身体需要一切有利条件来改善记忆能力。

喝足够的水和保持人体有足够的水分很重要，因为脱水真的会导致记忆力出现问题。

**2）锻炼身体**。如果您的医生说您可以进行锻炼，那么最好是制定一个锻炼计划：一个既有提高心率的运动，也有力量训练的计划。运动是最有益的健康习惯，也是经研究表明对大脑有益的习惯。运动不仅能让心脏和肌肉更强壮，还能在医学影像可见的程度，改变人的大脑结构。

**3）保持睡眠充足**。如果您睡眠不好，了解能让您睡得更好的方法，或者和您的医生谈谈。我喜欢这样比喻：睡觉的时候，有一辆环卫车将大脑中的"垃圾"搜集与清理掉；请不要让睡眠不足或睡眠质量差来耽误清理大脑垃圾的工作。现在也有研究证实了这一点。

**4）花时间与家人朋友在一起**。与朋友交往和交谈，多和人说说话。有研究表明，社交活动与较低的记忆力衰退的几率有关联，也就是说社交可以让记忆力保持得更好和更久。研究人员发现，社交活动多的人在记忆力测试中表现会更好。

**5）降低风险**。这是说不要做那些对身体有害、对心脏有害的事情。吸烟就是对身体和健康不利的行为。我们知道吸烟对我们的身体健康有害，但吸烟实际上也会影响我们的大脑健康。

健康的心脏对我们的大脑非常重要，这很容易理解。大脑需要从心脏泵出来的新鲜血液，所以心脏的健康很重要。血液将葡萄糖或血糖输送到大脑——它们是大脑的能量来源。所以，如果人的血糖有问题，血糖过高、过低，就会对大脑造成严重损害，导致记忆力问题。

**A. 戒烟**。如果您还在吸烟，请戒烟。另外，也不要和吸烟的人在一起，因为二手烟也是有害的。

**B. 糖尿病**。您检查过血糖吗？现在医学人员都知道糖尿病，甚至包括糖尿病前期（血糖水平上下波动，没有得到控制）都与老年痴呆症有关。所以请您减少食用加工的糖类食品。

**C. 高血压**。控制血压非常重要。道理很简单，大脑承受过多的压力可不是一件好事。

**D. 抑郁和焦虑**。研究表明，抑郁和焦虑的人更有可能出现记忆问题。医学人员还不知道确切的原因，但它意味着我们要认真对待这些情绪，在必要时寻求帮助。如果您现在有这类情绪上的困扰，是有许多解决方法的。

**E. 炎症**。体内的炎症对我们没有好处。头颈部的炎症（称为血脑屏障）后果尤其严重。如果血脑屏障，也就是脊髓液连通大脑的那道"关卡"发生炎症，它就会比正常状态下，更容易有其它物质进入大脑，包括破坏大脑的物质。所以，您要照顾好自己的身体，包括定时看牙医预防牙龈疾病（实质也是身体的一种炎症）。

**6. 锻炼您的大脑**。就像我们的身体需要锻炼一样，我们的大脑也需要锻炼。给大脑安排一些有挑战性的活动，可以是您喜欢的任何事。比如游戏、玩拼图、阅读、学习新事物，或是其它爱好。也可以做志愿者去帮助他人，尤其是在您退休之后。

**7. 减轻压力**。长期的压力实际上会损害大脑，使学习变得困难，并导致记忆力问题。冥想、瑜伽和其他身心活动已经被证明可以改善许多大脑问题。冥想和瑜伽甚至可以改变我们的大脑结构，缓减大脑记忆区域的炎症。

**8. 音乐**。我知道您非常喜欢音乐，所以请尽情欣赏您最喜欢的音乐或者去唱歌吧。我认为这会让您更快乐。有一些新的研究也表明音乐对大脑的不同部分有着刺激作用。

**9. 爱和感恩**。祈祷并心存感激。就像您一直教导的那样，我现在同样建议您这么做。或许我还可以在这里加上冥想（禅修），无论您做了什么，请坐下来做一个深呼吸，上帝与您同在。我不确定在这一点上是否有研究支持，但我想这也许是最好的建议了。

这些都是关于大脑健康的一些建议。您可以选择对您有用的方式。

### 去看医生或去医院

好了，现在让我们谈谈去看医生或去医院检查您的记忆问题。这是非常重要的。在这一部分我将说一些非常专业的内容，因为您和我都在医院工作过，我想您会希望了解更多有用的细节。如果您对我的某些说法不明白，请让您的医生解释一下。

### 看医生

务必在看医生时**有人随您一同前往**。

这是很重要的。如果您能找一个了解您、熟悉您的人（比如妈妈）、能证实您的记忆问题的人，让这个人告诉医生需要认真对待您的问题，这会非常有用。妈妈（或者随您见医生的任何人）也可以在边上帮您做笔记，这样您只要用心听医生说话就行了。

**如果您记忆有问题或有轻度认知障碍，医生需要做哪些检查？**

医生需要了解您的生活的下列方面（您可以做笔记或在见医生前打印这份清单）：

1. 记忆和认知功能上的变化，何时开始、发生了什么变化、记忆有问题的实际例子。

2. 日常活动能力的变化。包括日常起居活动或者你如何管理你的一天以及您在处理财务和钱上面遇到的困难。

3. 您的饮食和饮水状况怎么样？记住人体脱水（没有喝足够的水）也可以导致记忆力上的问题。

4. 当前服用的处方和非处方药。包括维他命和营养品。

5. 与大脑有关的症状，如听觉、视力、语言、睡眠、行走、肢体麻木或身体任何部位的刺痛。

6. 与心脏健康有关的症状。大脑要得到足够的血液，从心脏到大脑的血液流动正常，大脑能够从血液中得到适量的血糖（葡萄糖）。这点是我在前面提到过的，如果您有任何症状，如高血压、糖尿病前期或糖尿病，或任何心脏问题，包括心率不齐，请准备好与医生讨论这些症状。

7. 心理健康或情绪问题，如抑郁、焦虑、行为或性格的变化，这些都可能导致记忆力问题。

8. 家族病史。医生还可能询问您的家族病史。据我所知，我们很幸运，没有家人有过什么严重的记忆力受损或老年痴呆的疾病。但是，父亲，如果您知道我们的家族中有人有这些病史，请告诉医生。

**医生或医务人员还会对您进行身体检查，及对您进行神经上的医学检查。**

父亲，我想您应该去看医生。让医生问您一些问题，为您做些检查，以确定您的健康状况。

**血液检测**

父亲，在您这个年纪来说，因为记忆出现问题而进行血液检查是很正常的。因为您的记忆问题可能是某种身体状况造成的，也可能只是由于缺乏某类维生素或矿物质而造成的。

这些是我所了解的您应该做的检查（至少要做这些，如果您有医疗保险的话）：血液检测包括一个完整的生化检测项目清单，至少要包括：全血细胞计数、电解质项、血葡萄糖浓度、钙含量、甲状腺功能项、血液内铁、维生素 B12 和叶酸的含量。当然医生可能还会提议增加其它血液检测的项目。

对您的血液进行这些项目的检测，其目的是识别那些可逆的轻度认知障碍、感染、肾的问题、身体内镁元素太多或太少、钙元素过多或过少、血糖水平（高血糖）、甲状腺问题、维生素和营养问题（维生素 B12、铁或叶酸缺乏），这些原因导致的认知障碍是可以恢复的。考虑到我们美国人的饮食习惯，如果您有上述生理指标的异常，这并不奇怪（开玩笑的）。

其它的生化检测，可能包括对肾功能和肝功能的检查。此外，莱姆病、梅毒和艾滋病也是认知障碍的罕见原因。但您要知道，除非您对医生说了什么，否则医生是不会想到进行这些检测的，也不会进行其它性病的检测（我想您现在在笑）。

现在同样有对睡眠呼吸暂停的检查，如果您晚上睡觉打鼾或常常呼吸困难，这些健康问题也可能影响您白天的专注力和您的记忆力。

**专业的用药检查，为什么？**

父亲，因为您是药剂师，我想您明白为什么您需要进行专业的用药检查。用药检查对记忆力有问题的人尤其重要。某些种类的药物和药物的组合可能会导致记忆问题和认知障碍，所以您当前服用的所有处方药、非处方药物和维生素都必须告诉医生，并进行用药检查。

您现在可能不需要知道这些，但是最有可能导致认知障碍的药物包括抗胆碱能药、鸦片类、苯二氮卓类和非苯二氮平类安眠药（如唑吡坦）、地高辛、抗组胺药、三环类抗抑郁药、肌肉松弛药和抗癫痫药物。更年期的激素疗法（单用雌激素或雌激素加黄体酮组合使用）已被证明会增加轻度认知障碍或老年痴呆的风险。此外，用于治疗高血压的降血压药物、用于血糖问题（包括低血糖、高血糖、糖尿病前期、高血糖引起的糖尿病前期和糖尿病）的药物，也都可能导致患者的认知障碍。

## 记忆力测验或认知测验

我希望有人给您做记忆力的测验或认知测试。医护人员也会做一些基本的记忆力或认知测试，这些测验大概会耗时 10-20 分钟。医生可能会使用多种不同的测试方法，他可能会使用蒙特利尔认知评估量表（MoCA）、简易智力状态评估量表（Mini- cog），或者我比较喜欢的 3MS（改良简易精神状态测试）。如果医生想要做更多的检查，那是好事，因为您可以得到更好更全面的检查。这些检查结果会很有用。如果医生在半年或一年后再找您谈话，您将能够看到您的记忆发生了什么改变或是保持了不变。第一次记忆力测验会被当做"基准"，后续测验将与这一基准对照。我要再说一次，亲爱的爸爸，这些测验都是很有用的。

## 大脑医学影像扫描：检查您的大脑

父亲，您知道现在的医学技术非常发达。如果您可能有记忆力的问题，那么医生很可能会建议您做一些脑部扫描——或者说生成您大脑的影像。面对医生的这类建议，请您放心的接受。这些扫描是无痛的，您只需要静静地躺在机器里 30 - 45 分钟，然后医生就会拍摄您大脑的影像。

大脑医学影像扫描有好几种不同技术。磁共振成像（MRI）和 CT 扫描（计算机断层扫描）都是很好的检查手段。但通常医生只建议病人接受一种检测，当然也可能进行多种方式的检测。

为什么医生要求做这种脑部扫描？他们的目的是检查脑部是否有肿块、出血或感染。由于所有人的大脑都会萎缩，医生也会查看"大脑总体积"，以确定大脑的萎缩状况，是否与您的年龄相符，没有出现萎缩过快。他们还会查看大脑的其他方面或大脑结构的变化，确认是否有任何异常。

像我之前提到的那样，现在进行这些检测和其他检测，可以作为一种数据"基准"。如果您在一两年后仍然有记忆问题，并且这些问题不能自行改善，医生可以再做这样的检测，然后他们可以将结果与之前的"基准"进行比较，从而得到有意义的信息。

另一个进行脑部成像的好处是，**如果您曾经中风、不自觉的中风（自身没有觉察到的中风）或短暂性脑缺血发作（TIA）**，也可能会有记忆受损，但这是可以部分恢复或全部恢复到之前的功能和记忆力状态的。很多时候，这类中风是可以在大脑影像上看到的。这是很重要的，因为您需要去找心脏病医生或神经科医生，寻找方法缓解或消除这些健康问题，确保您不再发生中风，而这些影像对这些医生也是有用的。

**从上面这些检查、测验中，我们能得到什么？**

如果发现有任何显著的结果或现象，那么医生将尝试治疗这些病症，观察您的记忆力能否得到改善。医生还会与您和家人（或与您一起去看医生的人）讨论在轻度认知障碍上的发现。

不管怎样，医生会要求六个月后再次复查。因此，大约每六个月安排一次复查是非常重要的。通过复查，医生可以观察您的记忆与认知功能和需求的变化（包括改善）。

**转诊（如有必要）**

父亲，如果您的记忆力出现了严重的问题，我希望您的基本的医疗服务人员和医生能够将您转到更专业的专家那里。因为专业领域的医学专家能知道如何更好治疗，他们知道要检测什么，也知道什么会对您有帮助。这类专家通常是神经科的医生或老年医学的专家（专门为老年人提供医疗服务的人）。

**轻度认知障碍的确诊**

**轻度认知障碍（MCI）的确诊需要哪些必要的信息和达到哪些标准？**

要确诊轻度认知障碍，医生需要下面这些信息（记住这些确诊标准可能会随时变化）：

1. 医生或其他认识的人（经过观察）对疑似患者的思维能力（认知能力）的改变表示忧虑。

2. 在一个或多个认知领域上发现了认知障碍的"客观的证据"（见上面的医学检测），包括记忆力、执行功能、专注力、语言或视觉空间技能。

3. 在身体功能上的独立能力（虽然一个正常人在日常生活和使用工具的活动中，也有低效或出错的情况）。

4. 没有证据表明有明显的社会或职业功能障碍依据（如：没有痴呆症）。

我希望您能看到上面列出的症状，它们并不是严重的问题，但在医学上现在都是轻度认知障碍迹象。

上面是有关轻度认知障碍的一些细节和基本的医疗人员或医生会帮助您的事情。最后，我想和您谈谈离开医生的办公室后，您可以做的有助于您的记忆能力的其他事情。

请与您的基本的医疗服务人员或全科医生预约。如果您愿意，还可以先行填好自检日志和表单（为期 **10** 周），并把它们交给医生。您可以自己填写下面的自检日志和表单，但您身边有人帮您做更好。也许妈妈可以帮您填

写，或者我可以在电话里帮您填写。如需要我的帮忙，请告诉我。

我希望这封信对您有帮助。这是一封很长的信，但是我想让您知道这些信息，这些信息是我的专业领域内的东西。爸爸，我就在您身边，随时准备接您的电话。

我爱你，爸爸！我为您祈祷，愿上帝赐您健康、幸福与宁静。

永远爱你，

塔拉·罗丝

DEAR DAD, CAN WE TALK ABOUT YOUR MEMORY?

# Am I Having Memory Problems or Is This Normal?

## Worksheet
## 我是否出现了记忆上的问题？这是正常的吗？
## 自检表单

在去看医生或去医院之前，请将这份表单填好。然后带着这份表单去看医生。，现在的医生很忙，至少不会像以前的医生一样有很多时间来帮助每一位病人。，在与医生会面的有限时间内，提供给他/她这张表将对你和医生都有很大的帮助。

Your name: 您的姓名：

_____

Doctor/Health Care Provider: 医生、医疗机构：

_____

Appointment. Date: 预约的日期、时间：

_____

Doctor's/Provider's Phone Number: 医生或医疗机构的电话：

_____

**I have concerns about my memory.   I've written some notes and filled out this form about my memory concerns. Would you like me to read my notes? You can make a copy if you like.** 我担心自己的记忆力出现了问题。我已经写了一些东西并填好了这份表单，上面有关于我的记忆问题的一些信息。请您看看这些信息，如果需要可以复印一份。

**MEMORY: I am concerned about these things and I would like to know if this is normal or not:** 关于记忆：我对发生在我身上的一些事情很担心，我想知道它们是不是正常的？

---

# DEAR DAD, CAN WE TALK ABOUT YOUR MEMORY?

I am concerned about my memory, when I: 当我：

_____

的时候，我担心自己的记忆出现了问题。I am also concerned about my memory, when I 当我：_____

的时候，我也担心自己的记忆出现了问题

Another memory concern I have is: 此外，当我

_____

的时候，我也担心自己记忆出现了问题

Does anything make the memory problems worse or better? Are the memory concerns all the time or just sometimes (and when)? 什么会让我的记忆变好或变坏？这些记忆问题是总是有的还是偶尔才会发生的（什么时候会发生）？

    1. _____

    2. _____

These memory concern affect my day-to-day life by: 这些记忆问题会通过以下方式影响我的日常生活：

    1._____

    2._____

Medications, other physical problems: **药物和其它身体上的问题：**

_____

Mental health or well-being problems: 精神健康或情绪问题：

☐ Anxious or Anxiety 紧张或焦虑   ☐ Sadness or Depression 悲伤或抑郁

_____

Other problems in your life (short list) (changes or things/events that are stressful or not easy to deal with): 我生活中的其它问题（简单罗列出来）（变化或者是感到压力和难以处理的事情）：

_____

**Here are some things you may want to say to your doctor/health care professional at your appointment:** 下面是就诊时您可能想告诉医生或医护人员的其它事情：

"Can you do a memory screening test for me? Either at this appointment or at another appointment? I hear it only takes 10-15 minutes and I would like to know if there is a possible problem." "您能帮我做个记忆力测试吗？" 在这次或者在下次就诊时进行？我听说只需要 10-15 分钟，然后我想通过这个测试看看自己的记忆是否存在问题。"

"If it seems there might be a problem or a possible question about my memory, I would like some blood work to be done to make sure I don't have any causes of memory problems that are reversible, like a vitamin deficiency. Here is a letter my daughter wrote that lists the kinds of blood work that I may need."
"如果我的记忆力可能出现了问题，我希望做血液检查，以确定我的记忆问题是否是可逆的（不是病），比如维生素缺乏而导致记忆力下降。这是我女儿写的一封信，里面列出了我可能需要做的各种血液检查项目。"

"Can you also check my medications to make sure there aren't any interactions?" "您可以帮我检查一下我服用的药物，来确认这些药物是否与我的记忆问题有任何关联吗？"

DEAR DAD, CAN WE TALK ABOUT YOUR MEMORY?

## Am I Having Memory Problems

## A 10-Week Journal

我是否出现了记忆上的问题
为期 10 周的自查日志

Week: 周次：☐ 1　☐ 2　☐ 3　☐ 4　☐ 5　☐ 6　☐ 7　☐ 8　☐ 9　☐ 10

Today's date is: 今天的日期是：＿＿＿＿＿＿＿＿＿＿＿＿＿＿＿

☐ Monday 星期一　☐ Tuesday 星期二　☐ Wednesday 星期三

☐ Thursday 星期四 ☐ Friday 星期五　☐ Saturday 星期六　☐ Sunday 星期日

Big and small activities of the week or day: 本周或本天的大小活动：

＿＿＿＿＿＿＿＿＿＿＿＿＿＿＿＿＿＿＿＿＿＿＿＿＿＿＿＿＿＿

## Keeping Track of What I Am Forgetting

持续记录我忘记了什么

**My Memory issues/Forgetfulness this week:** 我的记忆力问题/我这周忘记了什么：

Did I forget something or have concerns about my memory today?

今天我是否已忘记了一些事，或今天我的记忆是否出现了状况？

☐ Yes 是　　☐ No 否　　☐ Maybe 可能有

**This week, did I forget or have trouble with:** *(check if you had problems)* 本周，我是否忘记了什么或在下面的事物上有麻烦：（勾选发生的事情）

**Forgetfulness:** 忘记了：
☐ Names 人的名字 ☐ Keys 钥匙 ☐ Wallet/bag/money 钱包、包、钱
☐ Cell phone 手机 ☐ What I wanted to say 我想说的事情
☐ Something else important 其它重要的事情 _____

**Location:** 位置、地点：
☐ Forgot day of the week 忘记今天是星期几
☐ Forgot where I was 忘记我在哪里

**Felt confused**: 感到困惑：
☐ What was I about to do 我接下来要做什么
☐ How to do something I normally do 如何按平时的方式做某件事

**Lost:** 迷路：
☐ Couldn't remember how to get somewhere 不记得如何去哪个地方

**Basics**: 基本的：
☐ Problem getting dressed 穿衣服上遇到了问题
☐ How to cook or get a meal 如何做饭
☐ How to pay a bill 如何付款

**What did I have problems with?** 我在哪方面出现了记忆力相关的问题？

_____

☐ I had memory problems but I don't remember what they were 我有记忆力的问题，但我不记得相关的问题是什么了。

# Am I Taking Care of my Brain Health?

## 我是否有在很好地照料我的大脑健康?

## A 10-Week Journal 为期 10 周的自检日志

Week: 周次： □ 1  □ 2  □ 3  □ 4  □ 5  □ 6  □ 7  □ 8  □ 9  □ 10

Today's date is: 今天的日期是： _____

□ Monday 星期一  □ Tuesday 星期二  □ Wednesday 星期三

□ Thursday 星期四  □ Friday 星期五  □ Saturday 星期六  □Sunday 星期日

Big and small activities of the week or day: 本周或本天的大小活动：

---

### Keeping Track of Healthy Brain Health 持续记录我的大脑健康状态

**Brain Health:** □ **Today I:**  □ **This week I:**

大脑健康： □ 今天，我： □ 这一周，我：

1. Drank enough water and made sure I was hydrated? 喝足够的水，确保自己身体内水分足够？
   □ Yes是  □ No 否  □ Maybe/Somewhat 也许

2. Ate healthy? 吃得健康吗？
   □ Yes是  □ No 否  □ Maybe/Somewhat 也许

3. Took my medication and/or vitamins for the day? 今天我服药了吗？和（或）服用维生素了吗？
   □ Yes是  □ No 否  □ Maybe/Somewhat 也许

---

4. Had enough / good sleep last night? 昨天晚上我睡得好、睡眠时间够么？
    ☐ Yes是    ☐ No 否    ☐ Maybe/Somewhat 也许

5. Had stress? 我是否感到压力？
    ☐ Yes是    ☐ No 否    ☐ Maybe/Somewhat 也许

    Managed the stress well? 我能否很好地管理这些压力？
    ☐ Yes是    ☐ No 否    ☐ Maybe/Somewhat 也许

6. Did body exercise (walk, aerobics, etc.)? 我锻炼身体了吗（走步、有氧运动等）？
    ☐ Yes是    ☐ No 否    ☐ Maybe/Somewhat 也许、

7. Had some kind of brain exercise? 我是否做了大脑的脑力活动？
    ☐ Yes是    ☐ No 否    ☐ Maybe/Somewhat 也许、

8. Had social time / time with family or friends? 我是否花时间社交或者与家人和朋友在一起？
    ☐ Yes是    ☐ No 否    ☐ Maybe/Somewhat 也许

9. Other ways to take care of brain health? 其它照顾大脑健康的方式？
_____
    ☐ Yes是    ☐ No 否    ☐ Maybe/Somewhat 也许

10. Other ways to take care of brain health? 其它照顾大脑健康的方式？
_____
    ☐ Yes是    ☐ No 否    ☐ Maybe/Somewhat 也许

**Arabic Language - اللغة العربية**

والدي العزيز, لقد أردت المزيد من المعلومات عن مخاوفك بشأن الذاكرة

هذا دليل إرشادي عن كل ما يجب عليك القيام به & مجلة صحية

تارا روز

جمة الدكتور /أحمد محمد رسلان

عن الترجمة: قام بالترجمة الدكتور / أحمد محمد رسلان وهو طبيب يعمل في مستشفى جامعة المنوفية بمصر وهو متخصص في التخدير ومهتم بالبحث العلمي وبأمراض الجهاز العصبي ولديه بحثان منشوران دوليًا ويقيم في مدينة أشمون بجمهورية مصر العربية.

---

### Dear Dad, Can We Talk About Your Memory?

### Wisdom on Brain Health

#### Tara Rose, Ph.D.

#### Ahmed Mohamed Raslan, MD

About Translation: Dr. Ahmed Mohamed Raslan is a physician in Menoufia University Hospital, Egypt. He specializes in anesthesia and interested in scientific research and neuro degenerative diseases with two international research publications. He lives in Ashmoun, Egypt.

---

DEAR DAD, CAN WE TALK ABOUT YOUR MEMORY?

## المقدمة

هذا خطاب لوالدي العزيز

أكتب ذلك لوالدي بعد زيارتي له حيث كان يعاني من بعض المشاكل في الذاكرة. وعلى الرغم من أن المشاكل التي يعاني منها ليست خطيرة جدًا ولكنه لاحظ وجود مشاكل في ذاكرته وقد قلقنا عليه بسببها. وهذا خطاب حب من ابنة إلى والدها لذلك فإنه يحمل طابعًا غير رسمي ولكنه يتضمن كذلك معلومات مفصلة وتقنية مناسبة لموضوع هذه المراسلة. لقد كنت أعمل أنا ووالدي في المستشفيات على مدار حياتنا المهنية وقد كان مجال عملي: تثقيف المرضى عن الخرف ومرض الزهايمر ولذلك فقد اردت أن أطلعه على آخر الأبحاث في هذا المجال.

وبينما اكتب هذا الخطاب إلى والدي فإنني لم أعطه له من قبل ـ فقد توفى قبل شهرين (بسبب آخر ليس له علاقة بمشاكل الذاكرة التي كان يعاني منها) عندما بدأت مشاركة هذا الخطاب وأوراق العمل حول موضوعات "هل أعاني من مشكلات في الذاكرة؟" و "هل أعتني بصحة عقلي؟" ولكنني أعتبر هذا الخطاب بمثابة تكريم لوالدي. لقد مضى ثلاثة أعوام الآن وقد قمت بتحديث المعلومات بينما أحتفظ بصوت ابنتي وهي تتحدث إلى والدي.

أود أن أنبه القارئ إلى أن هذا الخطاب تقني نوعًا ما لذا فقد يكون لك معرفة القليل عني وعن والدي: لقد كان والدي طبيبًا صيدليًا متقاعدًا ومديرًا لمستشفى. لذا فإن هذا الخطاب موجه لمن يملك مستوى عالٍ من فهم المشكلات الطبية بصفة عامة. أما بالنسبة لي فأنا أعمل كطبيبة نفسية متخصصة في علم الشيخوخة وأعمل في أحد مراكز أبحاث مرض الزهايمر في الولايات المتحدة الأمريكية. لذا فلدي خبرة جيدة في هذا المجال وأعمل على تثقيف الآخرين عن هذا المرض ولذا فقد أردت مشاركة هذه المعلومات مع والدي. والآن أود مشاركتها معكم. إذا كان هناك شيء ما لا يمكنكم فهمه فقوموا بتجاوزه الآن ومن ثم يمكنكم سؤال طبيبكم أو مقدم الخدمة الصحية الخاص بكم عنه لاحقًا.

برجاء ملاحظة أن هذا عبارة عن كتاب وأرجو منكم مشاركته مع آبائكم وأمهاتكم وفقًا لما ترونه مناسبًا. كما يمكنكم مشاركته كذلك مع أخوالكم وعماتكم وجميع أقاربكم وأصدقائكم أو أزواجكم.

أنصحكم كذلك باستخدام المعلومات المذكورة في هذا الخطاب ولكن لا تنسوا أنه يجب عليكم الذهاب إلى طبيب قبل كل شيء إذا كنتم تعانون من مشاكل في الذاكرة. برجاء أخذ هذا الخطاب والاستبيانات المرفقة

119

معكم أثناء الذهاب إلى الطبيب. لا تأخذوا محتويات هذا الخطاب كنصيحة طبية ولكن قوموا بقراءتها بعناية واهتموا بأنفسكم. لا تعتبر المشكلات الكبيرة في الذاكرة شيئًا طبيعيًا مع التقدم في السن ويوجد الكثير من الطرق لعلاج أعراض الذاكرة وحماية أنفسكم من الخرف وتأخير ظهور مشاكل الذاكرة إذا كنتم تعانون من أي مرض.

اعتنوا بأنفسكم,

تارا

120

## الأسئلة التي لديك حول مشاكل الذاكرة الأخيرة التي تعاني منها

والدي العزيز,

لقد قلت أنك كنت وما زلت تعاني من مشكلات في الذاكرة وأن لديك بعض الأسئلة التي تود معرفة إجابتها. أعتقد أن أفضل طريقة لكي أقدم إليك بعض النصائح هو عن طريق كتابتها لك في خطاب. أنت تعلم أنني أعمل في مجال أبحاث مرض الزهايمر ومشاكل الذاكرة ولذلك فلدي الكثير من النصائح لكي أقدمها لك. ولأنني ابنتك كذلك فإنني سأحرص على أن أقدم لك أفضل نصيحة ممكنة. لذلك أطلب منك أن تستمع لما سأقوله لك وأن تعلم أنه يأتي من صميم قلبي وأنني قد ركزت في نفس الوقت على الجانب الأكاديمي أكثر - بشكل محدود رغم ذلك - ولكن 30 عامًا من الخبرة في مجال أبحاث مرض الزهايمر ستكون نقطة انطلاق جيدة.

دعني ابدأ بعنوان "مشاكل الذاكرة" لقد سألتني ماذا سيفعل الطبيب إذا وجد أن مستوى ذاكرتك به مشكلة. حسنًا, من الممكن أن يقول لك أنك تعاني من "خلل إداركي بسيط". أعلم أن الكثير من الناس يقلق من الإصابة بمرض الزهايمر أو الخرف مع التقدم في السن. ومع ذلك, فإنني لا أتحدث في هذا الخطاب عن مرض الزهايمر أو الخرف ودعنا لا نتجاوز الأمر ونقفز إلى الاستنتاجات مباشرة لمجرد أنك تعاني ببساطة من بعض المشاكل في الذاكرة. بدلًا من ذلك أريد أن أتحدث إليك عن المعنى الحقيقي لمعاناتك من مشاكل في الذاكرة أو خلل إداركي بسيط. دعني أخبرك كذلك بما يقوله الباحثون والعاملون في المجال الطبي حاليًا عن الخلل الإداركي البسيط حتى تعرف آخر الأبحاث وأحدث المعلومات لكي تشعر ببعض الراحة عندما تعرف الحقائق التي ستساعدك على المضي قدمًا.

سأبدأ بتقديم نظرة عامة عن كل ما نعرفه حاليًا عن مشاكل الذاكرة البسيطة.

يعني الخلل الإداركي البسيط أنك تعاني من تغيرات ملحوظة في ذاكرتك وقدرتك على التفكير, كما أخبرتني بنفسك, ومع ذلك فإن هذه التغيرات غير خطيرة أو شديدة بدرجة كافية تستدعي حصولك على مساعدة من الآخرين لممارسة أنشطتك اليومية المعتادة. أحيانًا ما يعرف هذا المستوى من مشاكل الذاكرة كذلك باسم "الاضطراب العصبي الإدراكي البسيط ويعرف بأنه تناقص ملحوظ في القدرة الإدراكية أكثر من التغيرات الطبيعية التي تحدث في الشيخوخة. تذكر: أن ذلك لا يعتبر خرف أو مرض الزهايمر!

قبل أن أمضي قدمًا فيجب أن أخبرك عن تعريف الخرف ومرض الزهايمر حتى تعرف لماذا ذكرت أنك لا تعاني من أي من هذه المشكلات الخطيرة.

الخرف (وكان يعرف قديمًا بالعته أو الشيخوخة في بعض الأوقات) يعني المعاناة من مشاكل كبيرة وواضحة في الذاكرة. يتضمن الخرف مجموعة من الأعراض أو المشكلات التي يعاني منها المريض. وخاصة في شكل فقدان في القدرة على التفكير والتذكر والاستدلال المنطقي (الوظيفة الإدراكية) وأداء المهام اليومية

121

(القدرات السلوكية) بالقدر الذي يؤثر بشكل سلبي على الحياة والأنشطة اليومية للشخص. يتراوح الخرف في شدته من المراحل البسيطة عند بداية ظهوره حتى المراحل المتأخرة التي تؤثر بشكل خطير على الحياة اليومية للشخص ثم تأتي أخطر مرحلة وهي التي يحتاج الشخص المصاب بالخرف إلى الاعتماد على الآخرين بشكل كامل لأداء الأنشطة الأساسية لحياته اليومية.

ويعتبر مرض الزهايمر أحد الأسباب الرئيسة للخرف ولكنه ليس السبب الوحيد بالتأكيد. يتميز مرض الزهايمر بما يعرف باسم " اللُّويحات والتشابكات" التي يمكننا رؤيتها في المخ. تتكون هذه اللُّويحات من البروتينات التي تحل محل أجزاء من المخ بينما تحدث التشابكات عندما تبدأ الخلايا الهامة في الموت وترك مساحات فارغة في المخ. لذا فإن تشخيص الخرف يعني وجود أعراض بوجود فقدان كبير في الذاكرة ويعتبر مرض الزهايمر أحد الأسباب الممكنة للخرف. ويوجد كذلك العديد من الأمراض الأخرى التي تسبب الخرف.

تشخيص الخرف أو مرض الزهايمر يعني وجود حالة أكثر خطورة من الخلل الإدراكي البسيط.

أنا أحاول أن أطمئنك أبي العزيز ولكنني لست متأكدة إذا كان ما أقوم بتوضيحه لك سيجعلك تطمئن أكثر أم لا... هذه هي رؤية عامة عن الموضوع:

مستويات مشاكل الذاكرة:

المستوى الأولى: مشاكل منتظمة في الذاكرة مع التقدم في السن.

المستوى الثاني: مشاكل أكبر في الذاكرة تعرف باسم الخلل الإداراكي البسيط.

المستوى الثالث: مشاكل خطيرة في الذاكرة تسمى الخرف أو مرض الزهايمر.

هذا هو كل ما في الأمر ببساطة.

<u>التشخيص والعلاج وتوقعات سير المرض</u>

دعني أخبرك بما نعرفه نحن (الأطباء والباحثون) عن تشخيص وعلاج والتوقعات طويلة الأجل لسير نوع مشاكل الذاكرة التي تعاني منها وأقصد بذلك الخلل الإدراكي البسيط.

بشكل عام يمكننا أن نقول بأن نسبة 10% إلى 20% من الأشخاص الذين تتجاوز أعمارهم 65 عامًا أو أكثر يعانون من الخلل الإدراكي البسيط أو ما يعرف بالاضطراب العصبي الإدراكي البسيط. ونحن نعلم أن خطر حدوث هذه المشكلات يزيد مع التقدم في العمر وأن الرجال أكثر عرضة لخطورة التعرض لهذه المشاكل من النساء.

لذلك وعلى الرغم من أن الأشخاص الذين يعانون من الخلل الإدراكي البسيط يكونون أكثر عرضة لخطورة الإصابة بالخرف مقارنة بأي شخص آخر في الولايات المتحدة الأمريكية فإنه يوجد نطاق كبير إلى حد ما من تقديرات نسبة الخطورة (يتراوح من أقل من 5% حتى 20% كنسبة تحول سنوية) وفقًا لمجموعة الأفراد أو السكان محل الدراسة. فإذا تم تشخيص ما بالإصابة بالخلل الإدراكي البسيط فإن نسبة احتمال تطور الأمر وتشخيصه بالإصابة بالخرف يتراوح من نسبة أقل من 5% حتى نسبة 20% سنويًا. وهذا يعني أن بعض الأشخاص تتحسن حالته ونسبة منهم تبقى ذاكرته كما هي, بينما تسوء حالة الذاكرة في البعض الآخر. وكوني ابنتك فأنا أتمنى بالتأكيد أن تتحسن ذاكرتك. يوجد الكثير من الأشياء التي قد تؤثر على ذاكرتك لذلك فعليك بالعمل لكي تصحح حالة ذاكرتك وتعود إلى حالتها "المعتادة".

هناك عدد من الأسباب التي تؤدي إلى معاناة كبار السن من الخلل الإدراكي البسيط أو تجعلهم أكثر عرضة للإصابة بمشكلات في الذاكرة والتفكير وغيرها من المشكلات الأخرى بما في ذلك الشعور بالحزن أو الاكتئاب أو تناول العديد من الأدوية التي تتفاعل مع بعضها (تعدد الأدوية) أو المشكلات المتعلقة بالقلب وتدفق الدم في الجسم (عوامل الخطورة الوعائية القلبية غير المتحكم فيها). تحتاج إلى النظر وأخذ هذه الأشياء في الاعتبار بواسطة طبيبك أو مقدم الخدمة الصحية الخاص بك.

لذلك أبي العزيز فإذا كنت لا تهتم بحالتك الآن وكانت مشاكل الذاكرة التي تعاني منها قابلة للعلاج - فقد تسبب حدوث تغير دائم يجعل هذه المشاكل غير قابلة للعلاج - لذا فأرجو منك أن تعتني بنفسك وأن تذهب إلى الطبيب الآن!

كما ترى فإن أهم رسالة أود توصيلها إليك في هذا الخطاب هي أن تذهب للطبيب الخاص بك! وأن تعتني بنفسك وصحتك وسلامتك. الآن. أود أن أخبرك عن كيفية العناية بصحتك وذاكرتك وما الذي يجب عليك التفكير فيه عند زيارتك للطبيب.

ما الذي يمكنه مساعدتك الآن؟ اعتن بنفسك!!

ما الذي يمكنه مساعدتك بأفضل شكل ممكن ويقلل من خطورة مشاكل الذاكرة التي تعاني منها؟

أول شيء هو العناية بجسمك وعقلك. فكل منهما مرتبط بالآخر كما تعلم. إن العناية بأنفسنا يمكنه أن يحدث تغيرات إيجابية فسيولوجية على عقلنا. إنه أمر مذهل وقد أثبتت الأبحاث ذلك منذ وقت قريب. فهناك الكثير من الأبحاث الجديدة التي تدرس كيف يمكن لعادات صحية معينة (من الدراسات الإكلينيكية) أن تغير المخ وتحسن من الأداء العقلي. وقد أثبتت هذه الدراسات وقامت بقياس التغيرات التي تحدث في المخ من خلال فحص حالة مخ الأشخاص قبل بدء الدراسة ثم إجراء التجربة والدراسة بدمج النشاط \العادة الجديدة حتى نهاية الوقت المحدد للدراسة ومن ثم فحص حالة المخ مرة أخرى. يمكن للباحثين الآن رؤية كيف تنمو أجزاء هامة من المخ بالفعل أو تصبح حالتها الصحية أفضل. إن الأمر أشبه كما لو قمت بممارسة الرياضة ورفع الأثقال فسوف ترى أن عضلات يديك وقدميك ستكبر وتصبح أقوى. نفس الشيء يحدث مع المخ. ولكن

الفارق أننا لا يمكننا النظر مباشرة داخل المخ لكي نرى هذه التغييرات بدون استخدام التصوير الإشعاعي الذي يكلف آلاف الدولارات. ولأن الأمر يستغرق بعض الوقت لذاكراتنا لكي تتحسن فمن السهل أن نتخلى عن العادات والأنشطة الصحية. ولكن عندما نرى أن ذاكرتنا تصبح أفضل مع الوقت فإن الأمر يستحق القيام بعادات صحية جديدة والالتزام بها.

لن أكتب الكثير عن كل موضوع من قائمة النصائح التالية لأنه يوجد الكثير من الكتب التي تتحدث عن هذه الأمور. ولكنني أريد منك فقط أن تعرف الأنشطة الصحية الأساسية التي درستها هذه الأبحاث وأثبتت فائدتها للمخ. أعرف أن الأمر يحتاج لكثير من الجهد لتغيير هذه الأشياء وإضافة أنشطة جديدة إلى حياتنا. يوجد بعض الأمور التي يمكنني العمل عليها لذا يمكننا أن نقوم ببعض منها معًا رغم أننا لا نعيش في نفس المدينة.

1) تناول طعام صحي وشرب المياه بشكل كافٍ. تناول الأطعمة التي تنفع قلبك. يمكنك البحث عن أطعمة "صحية للقلب" على الإنترنت مثل الفواكه والخضروات وجميع البقول والمكسرات واللحوم خالية الدهن والسمك. وهناك الكثير للحديث عنه بخصوص " النظام الغذائي لمنطقة البحر المتوسط" يوجد بعض الدراسات التي اكتشفت أنه يمكن لفيتامينات وعناصر غذائية معينة أن تحسن من صحتك لذا سأخبرك المزيد عندما تنتهي هذه الأبحاث. ولكن الآن يمكنني القول بأن تناول أوميجا 3 الذي يوجد في الأسماك الزيتية يعد أمرًا هامًا للغاية ويعتبر أفضل مصدر مفيد للذاكرة وتشمل الأطعمة التي تحتوي على أوميجا 3 الأسماك السمينة مثل السالمون وسمك الماكريل والسردين. لا يوجد اي أبحاث أعرفها حول دور الأطعمة العضوية في مقابل الأطعمة غير العضوية ولكن نظرًا لأنك تعاني من مشكلات في الذاكرة بشكل ما فأنا أعتقد أنه يجب عليك إنفاق المزيد من الأموال على الأطعمة العضوية (الأطعمة التي تنمو بدون أي إضافات أو مبيدات حشرية) قدر الإمكان. وأنت \ نحن محظوظون بأنه يمكننا تحمل هذه التكلفة الإضافية وتذكر أن مخك يقول لك أنه يحتاج للمساعدة فلا تتناول أي أطعمة تحتوي على مواد كيميائية قد تؤذي الجسم.

كما أود أن أوضح لك نقطة أخرى لم يتم إجراء بحث كافٍ عليها وهي تناول فيتامينات متعددة ومكملات بشكل كافٍ (كما يصف لك مقدم الخدمة الصحية الخاص بك). فأرجو منك تناولها. فحتى إذا لم يكن لدينا أبحاث منتهية عن هذا الأمر حتى الآن فإن الجسم يحتاج لأي مواد قد يستفيد منها لمساعدة الذاكرة.

إن شرب مياة كافية والحفاظ على ارتواء الجسم يعد أمرًا هامًا لأن الجفاف يمكنه التسبب بمشكلات فعلية في الذاكرة.

2) التمارين الرياضية. إذا أخبرك طبيبك أنه يمكنك أداء تمارين رياضية فسيكون من الأفضل وضع خطة للتمارين الرياضية تتضمن الأنشطة التي ترفع من معدل ضربات قلبك والأنشطة التي تعتبر بمثابة تدريبات تقوية للجسم. تعتبر التمارين الرياضية أحد أكثر الأنشطة المدهشة وقد تضمن أحد الأبحاث التي أوضحت بالتصوير الإشعاعي أن التمارين الرياضية تغير بالفعل من تركيب المخ وليس من القلب والعضلات فقط.

3) احرص على النوم لفترات كافية. إذا كنت لا تحظَ بنوم كافٍ فقم بتجربة طرق للنوم بشكل أفضل أو تحدث إلى مقدم الخدمة الصحية الخاص بك. أنا أحب التشبيه الذي يصف النوم كما تأتي شاحنة القمامة لأخذ المخلفات والفضلات الباقية من مخك والتي لا يجب أن تبقى في المخ. لا تقم بإلغاء خدمة التخلص من القمامة من خلال عدم النوم. توجد العديد من الأبحاث التي تثبت ذلك أيضًا.

4) قم بقضاء وقت مع الأصدقاء والعائلة. حاول أن تكون شخصًا اجتماعيًا وأن تتحدث مع الآخرين. ادخل في محادثات مع أشخاص آخرين. توجد بعض الدراسات التي توضح أن النشاط الاجتماعي مرتبط بحدوث معدلات أقل من ضعف الذاكرة بمعنى أن ذاكرتك ستظل أفضل لفترة أطول. أثبت الباحثون أن الأشخاص الذين يكونون على اتصال أكثر بالآخرين يكون أداؤهم افضل في اختبارات الذاكرة.

5) المشاركة في تقليل الخطورة. يعني تقليل الخطورة التوقف عن فعل الأشياء التي نعرف أنها ضارة لجسمنا وليست جيدة لصحة قلبنا. ويعتبر التدخين مثالًا هامًا على هذه الأشياء. فنحن نعرف أنه ضار على صحتنا بشكل عام وقد يؤثر على المخ كذلك,

إن القلب الصحي هام جدًا لصحة المخ. وهذا أمر منطقي. فنحن نحتاج إلى توزيع الدم من القلب إلى المخ لذلك فإننا نحتاج إلى قلب صحي. ويحمل الدم الجلوكوز أو سكر الدم إلى المخ كذلك – لذا فهو يقوم بتوصيل الطاقة اللازمة إلى المخ. فإذا كان شخص ما يعاني من عدم وصول نسبة مناسبة من سكر الدم إلى المخ سواء كانت نسبة عالية جدًا أو قليلة للغاية أو إلى أجزاء الجسم الأخرى فإنها قد تلحق الضرر بالمخ وتسبب حدوث مشاكل في الذاكرة.

أ – أوقف التدخين إذا كنت تدخن مرة أخرى فأرجو منك التوقف عن التدخين. كذلك لا تجلس في مكان مع أي شخص يقوم بالتدخين لأن التدخين السلبي له آثار ضارة كذلك.

ب. السكر هل قمت بفحص نسبة السكر في دمك من قبل؟ لأننا نعرف الآن أن السكر وحتى مرحلة ما قبل السكر (عندما تكون مستويات السكر في الدم متذبذبة لأعلى ولأسفل وغير منتظمة) قد يكون لها علاقة بالإصابة بالخرف. وقم بتقليل السكر المعالج كذلك من فضلك.

ج. ضغط الدم العالي أو مرض ارتفاع ضغط الدم إن التحكم في ضغط دمك يعد أمرًا هامًا للغاية. فكر في الأمر – إن وجود ضغط أكثر من الطبيعي على المخ لا يعتبر أمرًا جيدًا له.

د. الاكتئاب والقلق أثبتت الأبحاث أن الأشخاص الذين يعانون من الاكتئاب والقلق يكونون أكثر عرضة للإصابة بمشاكل الذاكرة. ونحن لا نعرف بالتأكيد سبب ذلك ولكن يجب علينا التخلص من هذه المشاعر وطلب المساعد إذا لزم الأمر. يوجد الكثير من العلاجات إذا كنت تعاني من أي من ذلك الآن.

٥. الالتهابات  إن وجود التهابات في جسمنا يعتبر أمرًا غير جيد بالنسبة لنا. ويعتبر التهاب جزء الجسم حيث تقع الرأس على الرقبة (يعرف بالحاجز الدموي المخي) أمرًا سيئًا بشكل خاص.  ففي حالة حدوث التهاب في الحاجز الدموي المخي الذي يعتبر بمثابة "البوابة" الصغيرة حيث يدخل السائل الشوكي إلى المخ يؤدي إلى انفتاح هذا الحاجز بشكل أكثر من الطبيعي مما يعني أنه يمكن للمواد والأجسام الدخول إلى المخ وإلحاق ضرر كبير به. وهذا يعني أن العناية بجسمك بما في ذلك الذهاب إلى طبيب الأسنان لتتجنب أمراض اللثة (والذي يعد نوعًا من أنواع التهاب الجسم) يعد أمرًا هامًا.

6. قم بتدريب عقلك.  كما يحتاج جسمنا إلى التدريب فإن عقلنا يحتاج إلى تدريب كذلك.  وذلك من خلال تعريض عقلك لأنشطة فيها تحدي للعقل. كما تحب مثل الألعاب وحل الألغاز والقراءة وتعلم أشياء جديدة وممارسة هواية معينة.  وقد يكون ذلك التطوع لمساعدة الآخرين وخاصة بعد التقاعد عن العمل.

7. تقليل التوتر العصبي. يمكن للتوتر العصبي المزمن أن يدمر المخ ويجعل التعلم أكثر صعوبة ويسبب حدوث مشكلات في المخ.  وقد أظهر التأمل واليوغا وغيرها من الأنشطة الجسدية العقلية قدرتها على تحسين الكثير من المشاكل المختلفة.   كما يمكن للتأمل واليوغا تغيير تركيب مخنا وتقليل الالتهاب في مناطق المخ المسئولة عن الذاكرة.

8. الموسيقى. أنا أعلم أنك تحب الموسيقى كثيرًا لذا استمع إلى نغماتك أو أغنياتك المفضلة.  أعتقد أن هذا الأمر سيجعلك أقوى وأسعد وهناك بعض الأبحاث الجديدة التي تعرض كيف يمكن للموسيقى تحفيز مناطق مختلفة من الجسم.

9. الحب والامتنان. قم بالصلاة وأشكر الله.  لقد علمتني ذلك في حياتي وها أنا أذكرك به الآن؟  يمكنني أن أضيف التأمل هنا كذلك, كن مع الله, ومع ذلك فأنا واثقة أنك تفعل هذا.   ولكنني لست متأكدة من هذه النقطة الأخيرة فلم تتم أي دراسات أو أبحاث عنها ولكنني لا أتصور أي نصيحة أفضل منها.

يوجد الكثير من الأفكار للحفاظ على صحة المخ.  اختر ما يناسبك منها الآن.

الذهاب إلى الطبيب أو مقدم الرعاية

حسنًا لنتحدث الآن عن الذهاب إلى الطبيب أو مقدم الرعاية لفحص مشاكل الذاكرة التي تعاني منها.  وهذا يعد أمرًا هامًا جدًا.  وأسمح لي أن أكون تقنية أكثر في هذا الجزء ولكن نظرًا لأننا عملنا في المستشفيات لوقت طويل فأعتقد أنك تفضل معرفة مزيد من التفاصيل. إذا لم تستطع فهم بعض النقاط التي سأخبرك بها فيمكنك أن تطلب من الطبيب توضيحها لك.

بخصوص الموعد مع الطبيب

تأكد من اصطحاب شخص ما معك أثناء ذهابك إلى الطبيب.

هذه نصيحة هامة. وسيكون من الأفضل أن تصطحب شخصًا قريبًا منك يعرفك جيدًا (مثل أمي) بحيث يمكنه أن يؤكد مشاكل الذاكرة التي تعاني منها ويوصل الأمر بشكل أفضل للطبيب لكي يأخذ شكواك على محمل الجد. يمكن لأمي (أو أي شخص آخر يذهب معك) أن تأخذ بعض الملاحظات من كلام الطبيب بينما تكتفي أنت بالاستماع إليه فقط.

ما الذي يحتاج الطبيب إلى فحصه إذا كانت لديك مشاكل في الذاكرة أو تعاني من خلل إدراكي بسيط؟

يحتاج الطبيب إلى فهم الجوانب التالية من حياتك: (يمكنك أخذ ملاحظات و إعداد قائمة مسبقة بهذه الأمور قبل الذهاب إلى موعدك مع الطبيب)

1. التغيرات في الذاكرة \ الإدراك (متى بدأت وكيف تغيرت وأمثلة على مشاكل الذاكرة التي تعاني منها).

2. التغيرات في القدرة على القيام بالأنشطة اليومية. ويشمل ذلك أنشطة الحياة اليومية أو كيفية إدارتك ليومك والصعوبات التي قد تواجهها بما في ذلك العناية بالأمور المالية وإدارتها.

3. هل تأكل جيدًا وماذا عن شربك؟ نعم أقصد الماء والكحول! تذكر أن الجفاف (نتيجة عدم شرب الماء بشكل كافٍ) قد يسبب حدوث مشكلات في الذاكرة.

4. الوصفات الطبية التي تتناولها حاليًا والأدوية التي تأخذها بدون وصفة طبية ويشمل ذلك الفيتامينات والمكملات الغذائية.

5. الأعراض التي قد تتعلق بالمخ مثل: السمع والرؤية والحديث ومشاكل النوم والمشي والتنميل أو الشعور بوخز في أي جزء من الجسم.

6. الأعراض المتعلقة بصحة القلب ـ للتأكد من حصول المخ على التدفق المناسب للدم من القلب ومن ثم حصول المخ على الكمية المناسبة من الجلوكوز / سكر الدم. لقد ذكرت ذلك مسبقًا لذلك إذا كنت تعاني من أي أعراض مثل ارتفاع ضغط الدم أو مرض السكر أو مقدماته أو لديك أي مشكلات في القلب بما في ذلك وجود نبضات قلبية غير منتظمة فكن مستعدًا لمناقشة هذه الأمور مع طبيبك.

7. الصحة العقلية أو المشكلات النفسية مثل الاكتئاب أو القلق أو التغيرات في السلوك أو الشخصية والتي قد تكون سببًا في حدوث مشاكل الذاكرة.

8. التاريخ الأسري. سيود الطبيب كذلك معرفة بعض المعلومات عن تاريخنا الأسري.
على حد علمي فإننا محظوظون بعدم وجود تاريخ أسري بحدوث خرف أو مشاكل خطيرة في الذاكرة. ولكن إذا كنت تعلم أي شيء عن أسرتنا فقم بإخبار الطبيب على الفور.

سيود الطبيب أو مقدم الرعاية إجراء فحص جسدي وقد يقوم كذلك بفحص عصبي عليك. أريدك أن تمنح الطبيب الفرصة لتوجيه أسئلته إليك والقيام بجميع الفحص اللازم لمعرفة ما يحدث لك.

فحوصات الدم المعملية

يعتبر طلب تحاليل أو فحوصات معملية أمرًا طبيعيًا في عمرك لأن مشاكل الذاكرة قد تكون حالة مرضية أو مجرد نقص في فيتامين أو عنصر غذائي أدى إلى التأثير على الذاكرة.

وهذه هي قائمة التحاليل التي أعرف أن الطبيب سيطلبها منك على الأقل إذا كان لديك تأمينًا صحيًا: تشمل تحاليل الدم فحص أيضي كامل يشمل: صورة دم كاملة وأيونات وجلوكوز وكالسيوم ووظائف الغدة الدرقية ونسبة الحديد وفيتامين ب 12 والفولات. ولكن طبيبك قد يكون له جوانب أخرى يريد فحصها في دمك.

وسبب حاجتك إلى إجراء جميع هذه الاختبارات على دمك هو التعرف على الأشكال القابلة للعلاج للخلل الإدراكي البسيط بما في ذلك العدوى ومشاكل الكليتين وزيادة أو نقص الماغنسيوم بشكل كبير وزيادة أو نقص الكالسيوم ومستويات نسبة الجلوكوز في الدم (زيادة نسبة الجلوكوز) ومشاكل الغدة الدرقية ومشاكل الفيتامينات او المواد الغذائية (فيتامين ب 12 والحديد ونقص نسبة الفولات). ولن تكون مفاجأة إذا اكتشف أنك مصاب بأي شيء من هذه القائمة بفضل الطعام الأمريكي الذي تتناوله.

قد يطلب الطبيب كذلك فحص وظائف الكبد والكليتين. كما يعتبر كل من مرض لايم والزهري والإيدز أحد الأسباب النادرة لنقص الإدراك. ولكن اعلم أن الطبيب قد لا يبدأ بهذه الاختبارات أو يفحص وجود أمراض منتقلة جنسيًا ما لم تخبره بشيء ما (أنا أمزح معك هنا)

كما يوجد اختبار معملي كذلك لانقطاع النفس أثناء النوم أو عندما تقوم بإصدار صوت شخير أو تعاني من مشكلات مع التنفس بانتظام أثناء الليل مما قد يؤثر على قدرتك على التركيز والتذكر على مدار اليوم.

مراجعة فنية للأدوية: لماذا؟

تريد مراجعة فنية للأدوية. تدرك ذلك لكونك صيدلي, وهو أمر هام خاصة لمن يعانون من مشاكل في الذاكرة. يمكن أن تؤدي بعض فئات ومجموعات الأدوية إلى مشاكل في الذاكرة والخلل الإدراكي, لذا ينبغي مراجعة جميع الوصفات الحالية والأدوية بدون وصفات طبية والفيتامينات.

ربما لا تحتاج إلى معرفة ذلك الآن, لكن فئات الأدوية التي تؤدي غالبًا إلى خلل إدراكي تتضمن مضادات الكولين, الأفيونات, البينزوديازيبينات, و المنومات الغير بينزوديازيبينة (مثل زولبيديم), الديجوكسين, مضادات الهستامين, مضادات الاكتئاب ثلاثية الحلقات, باسطات العضلات الحركية ومضادات الصرع. تبين أن العلاج الهرموني (الإستروجين فقط أو الإستروجين والبروجستيرون) يزيد من نقطة النهاية المشتركة للخلل الإدراكي البسيط أو الخرف (ليس أنها تنطبق عليك حقًا, لكن ربما تجد الأمر مثيرًا للاهتمام). بالإضافة إلى ذلك, ربما يؤدي أي من الآتي إلى مشكلات إدراكية مثل الأدوية الخافضة لضغط الدم المرتفع (ارتفاع

ضغط الدم), مرض ضغط الدم المرتفع, ومشكلات سكر الدم مثل انخفاض أو ارتفاع سكر الدم, ومرحلة ما قبل السكري (نتائج ارتفاع سكر الدم), ومرض السكري.

اختبار الذاكرة أو الإدراك

نحتاج لشخص ما ليقوم بأداء اختبار الذاكرة أو الإدراك لك. سيقوم مقدم الخدمة الطبية أيضًا بإجراء اختبار بسيط للذاكرة والإدراك يستغرق حوالي 10-20 دقيقة. هناك عدد من الاختبارات المختلفة التي يمكن أن يستخدمها الطبيب ويمكن أن يختار منها تقييم مونتريال الإدراكي, أداة تقييم الإدراك الصغيرة, أو الاختبار المفضل لديّ وهو اختبار الحالة العقلية الصغير المعدل. إذا أراد الطبيب إجراء المزيد من الفحوصات, فقط كن سعيدًا لتلقي تقييم أفضل وأكثر شمولاً. ستساعدنا هذه النتائج كثيرًا. وإذا تحدث إليك الطبيب مرة أخرى خلال ستة أشهر أو سنة من الآن, ستستطيع أن تدرك إذا ما تغيرت ذاكرتك أو ما زالت على حالها. اختبار الذاكرة الأول لك يسمى "خط الأساس" وسيساعدنا كثيرًا.

اطلب فحوصات للمخ: تصوير المخ

أصبحت التكنولوجيا مذهلة الآن, وإذا اتضح أنك تعاني من أي مشاكل في الذاكرة, ربما يطلب الطبيب بعض الفحوصات أو الصور للمخ. من فضلك "وافق" على ذلك. لن تشعر بأي ألم, عليك فقط أن تستلقي لمدة 30-45 دقيقة في جهاز وسيلتقطون صورًا لدماغك.

هناك نوعان مختلفان للفحوصات التي يمكن إجراؤها على الدماغ. أشعة الرنين المغناطيسي أو الأشعة المقطعية والتي تسمى أيضًا الأشعة المقطعية الهيكلية وكلاهما جيدان. يطلب الطبيب عادة نوع واحد أو أكثر من الأشعة.

لماذا يقومون بهذه الاختبارات للدماغ؟ للتأكد من عدم وجود أي كتل أو نزيف أو عدوى. بما أن أدمغتنا جميعًا تضمر, سينظر الأطباء أيضًا إلى حجم الكتلة الكلية ليتمكنوا من تحديد إذا كان الفقدان أو الضمور يتناسب مع عمرك أم أكثر من ذلك. سيبحثون أيضًا عن أنواع أخرى من التغيرات الدماغية أو الهيكلية لاستبعاد وجود أي شئ غير معتاد.

من الجيد إجراء هذه الفحوصات وغيرها لتكون خط الأساس كما ذكرت سابقًا, وإذا ظلت مشاكل الذاكرة خلال عام أو عامين ولم تتحسن من تلقاء نفسها, ربما يطلب الطبيب فحوصات أخرى ويقارن فيما بينها.

وهناك سبب مهم آخر لتخضع لهذه الفحوصات, إذا أصبت بجلطة, جلطة صامتة (بمعنى أنك لا تدركها) أو نوبة إقفارية عابرة, ربما تصاب بفقدان الذاكرة لكن ربما تستعيد بعض أو جميع وظائف الذاكرة والإدراك السابقين. يحدث كثيرًا أن نتمكن من رؤية هذه الجلطات في أشعة المخ وهذا أمر مهم حينها لأنك تحتاج

129

إلى زيارة إخصائي قلب و مخ وأعصاب للتقليل أو الحد من هذه المشكلات الصحية - وضمان عدم تكرارها مجددًا!

ماذا نجد في نتائج التقييمات والاختبارات؟

إذا كانت هناك أي تغيرات كبيرة في النتائج, عندها سيحاول الطبيب معالجة هذه الأعراض أملًا في تحسن ذاكرتك.  سيريد الطبيب أيضًا مناقشة نتائج أشعة الرنين المغناطيسي معك ومع أفراد العائلة (أو من يذهب معك لزيارة الطبيب).

في كلتا الحالتين, سيريد الطبيب رؤيتك مجددًا بعد ستة أشهر.  لذا, من المهم الترتيب لموعد للمتابعة تقريبًا بعد ستة أشهر حتى يتمكن الطبيب من معرفة التغيرات (بما فيها التحسن) في وظائف الذاكرة والإدراك وكذلك معرفة احتياجاتك.

الإحالة, إذا كانت هناك حاجة إليه

إذا كنت تعاني من أي مشكلات خطيرة في الذاكرة, أريد من طبيب الرعاية الأولية أو مقدم الخدمة الصحية أن يقوم بإحالتك إلى مختص لأن الخبراء مهمون ويعلمون ما هي الفحوصات اللازمة وكذلك ما يمكنه أن يساعد.  سيكون هذا الشخص عادة إخصائي أعصاب أو كبار السن (يعمل مع البالغين الكبار).

تشخيص الاضطراب الإدراكي البسيط

ما هي المعلومات الضرورية أو المعايير اللازمة لتشخيص الخلل الإدراكي البسيط؟

هذه بعض المعلومات التي يستخدمها الطبيب لتشخيص الخلل الإدراكي البسيط, لكن ربما تتغير بعض المعايير مثل:

1. تعبير الشخص عن القلق بخصوص تغير في قدرات التفكير (الإدراك), أو من شخص قريب أو من الطبيب الملاحظ للشخص.

2. "دليل موضوعي" على الاضطراب (انظر الاختبارات السابقة) في إحدى المناطق الإدراكية أو أكثر متضمنة الذاكرة أو الوظائف التنفيذية أو الانتباه أو اللغة والمهارات البصرية الفضائية.

3. الحفاظ على الاستقلالية في القدرات الوظيفية (بالرغم من أن الشخص قد يصبح أقل كفاءة وأكثر عرضة للقيام بأخطاء في أداء الأنشطة واستخدام الأدوات اليومية من السابق).

4. عدم وجود دليل على اضطراب شديد في الوظائف الاجتماعية أو المهنية (عدم الإصابة بالخرف).

أتمنى أن تتمكن من رؤية هذه القائمة التي توضح بعض المشكلات, لكنها ليست كبيرة, وهي تمثل خلل الإدراك البسيط.

هذه بعض التفاصيل وما يمكن أن يقوم به مقدمو الخدمة الصحية أو الأطباء لمساعدتك. الآن أريد أن أتحدث إليك بخصوص بعض الأمور الأخرى التي يمكن أن تقوم بها بمجرد أن تغادر مكتب الطبيب لتساعد ذاكرتك بقوة.

من فضلك حدد موعدًا مع مقدم الخدمة الصحية أو الممارس العام, وإذا أردت, استخدم صحيفة العشرة أسابيع وأوراق العمل بالأسفل وأحضرهم للطبيب. يمكنك تعبئة الصحيفة وأوراق العمل بنفسك, لكن في بعض الأحيان قد يقوم بذلك بعض المقربين بشكل أفضل. ربما تستطيع أمي تعبئتها لأجلك, أو نستطيع أن نفعل ذلك سويًا على الهاتف. أخبرني فقط إذا احتجت لأي مساعدة.

أتمنى أن تجد ذلك مفيدًا. أدرك أن الخطاب طويل, لكن أردتك أن تكون على علم بهذه المعلومات فهذا مجالي. أنا بجانبك فلا تتردد في طلبي إذا احتجت لأي شيء.

أحبك يا أبي. أدعو لك دائمًا في صلاتي, ليمنحك الله الصحة والعافية والسلام.

لك كل حبي وأكثر,

تارا روز

# DEAR DAD, CAN WE TALK ABOUT YOUR MEMORY?

# Am I Having Memory Problems or Is This Normal?

هل أعاني من مشكلات في الذاكرة أم أن هذا طبيعي؟

## Worksheet ورقة عمل

Fill this out before going to your health care provider's office – and bring it with you to your appointment. Physicians don't have that much time, at least not like they did in the "old days" so it would help to fill this out before going to the appointment and then showing it to the doctor if you start to run out of time with him or her.

املأ هذه الاستمارة قبل زيارة مكتب مقدم الخدمة الصحية الخاص بك — وخذها معك في الموعد المحدد. لا يمتلك الأطباء الكثير من الوقت, على الأقل ليس كما كان الحال في السابق لذا سيساعد كثيرًا أن تملأها قبل الذهاب إلى الموعد وتريها للطبيب إذا كان الوقت على وشك النفاذ قبل الانتهاء من المقابلة معه أو معها

Your name: الاسم

_____

Doctor/Health Care Provider: الطبيب/ مقدم الخدمة الصحية

_____

Appointment. Date: تاريخ المقابلة

_____

Doctor's/Provider's Phone Number: رقم هاتف الطبيب/مقدم الخدمة الصحية

_____

**I have concerns about my memory.  I've written some notes and filled out this form about my memory concerns. Would you like me to read my notes? You can make a copy if you like.**

لدي بعض المخاوف بخصوص ذاكرتي وقمت بتدوين بعض الملحوظات وملأت هذه الاستمارة بخصوص قلقي عن الذاكرة. هل تريد مني أن أقرأ ملحوظاتي؟ يمكنني ترك نسخة لك إذا أردت

---

**MEMORY: I am concerned about these things and I would like to know if this is normal or not:** الذاكرة: أنا قلق بخصوص هذه الأشياء وأريد أن أعرف ما إذا كان ذلك طبيعيًا أم لا:

I am concerned about my memory, when I:          :أشعر بالقلق حيال ذاكرتي عندما

_____

I am also concerned about my memory, when I عندما شعر بالقلق أيضًا حيال ذاكرتي:

_____

Another memory concern I have is:          :مخاوف أخرى بخصوص الذاكرة مثل

_____

Does anything make the memory problems worse or better? Are the memory concerns all the time or just sometimes (and when)?

هل يوجد شئ ما يزيد أو يقلل من مشاكل الذاكرة؟ هل تشعر بالقلق بخصوص الذاكرة في كل الأوقات أم أحيانًا ومتى؟

     1. _____

     2. _____

These memory concern affect my day-to-day life by:

يمكن لهذه المخاوف تجاه الذاكرة أن تؤثر على مسار الحياة اليومية من خلال:

     1._____

     2._____

**Medications, other physical problems:**          الأدوية, المشكلات البدنية الأخرى

_____

Mental health or well-being problems:          مشكلات السلامة أو الصحة العقلية

_____

    □ Anxious or Anxiety          القلق أو التوتر

    □ Sadness or Depression          الحزن أو الاكتئاب

_____

Other problems in your life (short list) (changes or things/events that are stressful or not easy to deal with):          شكلات أخرى في حياتك (قائمة قصيرة) (تغيرات أو أشياء/ أحداث مثيرة للتوتر أو ليس سهلاً التعامل معها)

_____

_____

_____

**Here are some things you may want to say to your doctor/health care professional at your appointment:**

هنا بعض الأشياء التي ربما تريد قولها للطبيب أو مقدم الخدمة الطبية أثناء المقابلة :

"Can you do a memory screening test for me? Either at this appointment or at another appointment?  I hear it only takes 10-15 minutes and I would like to know if there is a possible problem."

هل يمكنك أن تقوم باختبار فحص للذاكرة من أجلي؟ سواء خلال هذه المقابلة أو في مقابلة أخرى؟ أعرف أن الأمر يتطلب حوالي 10-15 دقيقة وأريد أن أعرف إذا ما كانت هناك مشكلة؟:

"If it seems there might be a problem or a possible question about my memory, I would like some blood work to be done to make sure I don't have any causes of memory problems that are reversible, like a vitamin deficiency.  Here is a letter my daughter wrote that lists the kinds of blood work that I may need."

إذا كانت هناك مشكلة أو تساؤل بخصوص حالة ذاكرتي, أريد أن أخضع لبعض فحوصات الدم لضمان عدم وجود أي أسباب يمكن علاجها, مثل نقص الفيتامينات. هذا خطاب من ابنتي دونت فيه قوائم بالفحوصات الطبية التي قد أحتاج إليها:

"Can you also check my medications to make sure there aren't any interactions?"

هل يمكنك تفقد أدويتي لضمان عدوم وجود أية تفاعلات بينها؟

DEAR DAD, CAN WE TALK ABOUT YOUR MEMORY?

**هل أعاني من مشكلات في الذاكرة**

**صحيفة العشرة أسابيع**

الأسبوع:1 10□ 9□ 8□ 7□ 6□ 5□ 4□ 3□ 2□

تاريخ اليوم :

_____

السبت □الأحد □الإثنين □الثلاثاء □الأربعاء □الخميس □الجمعة □

الأنشطة اليومية أو الأسبوعية الكبيرة والصغيرة

_____

تعقب ما أنساه

أمور خاصة بذاكرتي/النسيان هذا الأسبوع:

هل نسيت شيئًا ما أو لديك قلق بخصوص ذاكرتك اليوم؟

□ نعم      □ لا      □ ربما

اليوم, هل نسيت أو عانيت من مشكلة في الذاكرة: (تفقد إذا كنت تعاني من مشكلات )

( النسيان ):

□أسماء      □ مفاتيح      □محفظة / حقيبة / نقود      □ هاتف جوال

□ ما كنت أريد قوله

□شئ آخر هام _____

الموقع:

□ نسيت يوم الأسبوع      □نسيت أين كنت

# DEAR DAD, CAN WE TALK ABOUT YOUR MEMORY?

شعرت بالاضطراب:

☐كيف أفعل شئ ما اعتدت على فعله     ☐ما الذي كنت على وشك فعله

التوهان:

☐لم أستطع تذكر كيفية الوصول إلى مكان ما

الأساسيات:

☐كيفية طهو وجبة أو الحصول عليها     ☐مشكلة في ارتداء الملابس

☐كيفية دفع فاتورة

ما المشكلات التي عانيت منها؟

_____

☐عانيت من مشكلات في الذاكرة لكن لا أتذكر أين كانت

**هل أعتني بصحة عقلي؟**

**صحيفة العشرة أيام**

الأسبوع:1 10□ 9□ 8□ 7□ 6□ 5□ 4□ 3□ 2□

تاريخ اليوم :

_____

السبت □الأحد□ الإثنين □ الثلاثاء □ الأربعاء □ الخميس □ الجمعة □

الأنشطة اليومية أو الأسبوعية الكبيرة والصغيرة

_____

مراقبة صحتي العقلية

الصحة العقلية: □ اليوم: □ هذا الأسبوع: هل:

1. شربت كمية كافية من الماء وتأكدت من حصولي على كفايتي منه؟

نعم □   لا □   ربما \ إلى حد ما □

2. تناولت طعامًا صحيًا؟

نعم □   لا □   ربما \ إلى حد ما □

3. تناولت دوائي و/أو فيتاميناتي لليوم؟

نعم □   لا □   ربما \ إلى حد ما □

4. حصلت على نوم جيد/ كافي الليلة الماضية؟

نعم □   لا □   ربما \ إلى حد ما □

139

5. عانيت من التوتر العصبي؟

☐ نعم    ☐ لا    ☐ ربما \ إلى حد ما

تمكنت من التعامل جيدًا مع هذا التوتر العصبي؟

☐ نعم    ☐ لا    ☐ ربما \ إلى حد ما

6. قمت بالتمارين الرياضية (المشي, التمارين الهوائية وغيرها)؟

☐ نعم    ☐ لا    ☐ ربما \ إلى حد ما

7. قمت بأداء بعض التمارين العقلية؟

☐ نعم    ☐ لا    ☐ ربما \ إلى حد ما

8. حظيت بوقت اجتماعي / مع العائلة أو الأصدقاء؟

☐ نعم    ☐ لا    ☐ ربما \ إلى حد ما

9. طرق أخرى للعناية بصحة المخ؟

_____

☐ نعم    ☐ لا    ☐ ربما \ إلى حد ما

10. طرق أخرى للعناية بصحة المخ؟

_____

☐ نعم    ☐ لا    ☐ ربما \ إلى حد ما

## Hindi Translation - हिंदी में अनुवाद

प्रिय पापा,

यह पत्र में आपको यादशक्ति को लेकर आपकी जो चिंता है,

उसपर ज़्यादा जानकारी देने के लिए लिख रही हूँ।

कर्म मार्गदर्शिका एवं स्वास्थ्य पत्रिका।

तारा रोज़

आदित्य चाचाड

---

### Dear Dad, Can We Talk About Your Memory?

### Wisdom on Brain Health

### Tara Rose, PhD

### Aditya Chachad, BSSM, MPH

About the Translator: Aditya Chachad holds a Bachelors of Medicine and Bachelors of Surgery from Maharashtra University of Health Sciences, India. He also holds a Masters in Public Health from University of Southern California, Los Angeles. He has over 10 years of experience in clinical research in various clinical specialties including neurological and behavioral health, pediatrics and cardiovascular diseases.

DEAR DAD, CAN WE TALK ABOUT YOUR MEMORY?

# परिचय

यह पत्र प्रिय पापा के लिए है।

मेने अपने पिताजी को उनसे मिलने के बाद यह लिखा था, क्यूँकि उन्हें याददाश्त को लेकर कुछ दिक़्क़तें थीं। दिक़्क़तें ज़्यादा गम्भीर नहीं थी, पर उन्होंने इन दिक़्क़तों को महसूस किया था, जिसकी वजह से हम चिंतित थे। यह एक प्यार भरा पत्र है जोकि एक बेटी ने अपने पिताजी को लिखा है। इसी वजह से यह अनौपचारिक भाषा में लिखा गया है, लेकिन इसमें विस्तृत एवं तकनीकी जानकरियाँ हैं जो कि इस तरह के पत्र-व्यवहार से पायी जा सके। में और मेरे पिताजी, हम दोनो आजीवन अस्पताल में काम करने वाले व्यवसायी रह चुके हैं, और यह क्षेत्र में मेरी विशेषज्ञता थी: स्मृतिभ्रंश एवं अलज़ाइमर रोग (भूलने के रोग) की पढ़ाई, और इस वजह से में उन्हें इससे जुड़ी नवीनतम शोध के बारे में बताना चाहती थी।

जबकि यह पत्र मेने अपने पिताजी के लिए लिखा था, में उन्हें यह कभी दे नहि पायी, क्योंकि वह कुछ महीनो बाद गुज़र गए।(जिसका कारण उनकी यादशक्ति की तकलीफ़ नहि थी।) जब मेने इन पत्र और कार्यपत्रकों को पहली बार सांझा करना शुरू किया: "क्या मुझे याददाश्त की दिक़्क़त है?" और "क्या मैं अपनी मानसिक स्वास्थ्य की देखभाल कर रहा हूँ?", यह मुझे अपने पिताजी का मान रखने के तरीक़े की तरह प्रतीत हुआ। अब तीन साल बीत चुके हैं और मेने इस तकलीफ से जुड़ी पुरानी तथा नवीन जानकारियों को बनाए रखते हुए, अपने पत्र में एक बेटी की आवाज़ तथा अपने पिताजी के प्रति उसकी भावनाओं को बनाए रखा है।

143

में इस पत्र को पढ़ने वाले शक्स को यह चेतावनी देना चाहती हूँ कि यह पत्र काफ़ी हद तक तकनीकी है, तो आपके लिए मेरे और मेरे पिताजी के संदर्भ में कुछ बातें जानना फ़ायदेमंद रहेंगी। मेरे पिताजी एक सेवानिवृत्त फ़ार्मासिस्ट एवं अस्पताल के वरिष्ठ प्रबंधक थे, और इस कारण, एक बड़े स्तर पर कहा जाना चाइए की, 'यह पत्र किसी ऐसे व्यक्ति के लिए लिखा गया है जिसे चिकित्सक मसलों की उच्च स्तर पर समझ हो।' में एक नैदानिक मनोविज्ञानि हूँ जिसने जराविज्ञान (वृधवस्था और उसके रोगों का अध्ययन) किया है, और में एक अलज़ाइमर रोग अनुसंधान केंद्र (ADRC), युनाइटेड स्टेट्स, मे काम करती हूँ। इस कारणवश मुझे इस क्षेत्र का विशेषज्ञान है। दूसरों को शिक्षित करने के लिए, यह मेरा क्षेत्र है, और इसी वजह से में उन्हें यह जानकारी पारित करना चाहती थी। और अब आप को कर रही हूँ। अगर कुछ ऐसा हो जोकि आपके समझ ना आए, तो आप कृपा कर उसे फिलहाल के लिए वहीं छोड़कर आगे बढ़ जाइए, और बाद में आप अपने चिकित्सक या स्वास्थ्य देखबाल प्रदाता से उस बारे में सदा ही जानकारी हासिल कर सकते हैं।

कृपा कर ये जानें कि यह एक किताब है। कृपा कर इसे आगे अपने अभिभावकों के साथ ज़रूरत समझने पर सांझा करें। इसे आप आपके भाई-बहन, अंकल, आंटी, दोस्त एवं अपने पति या पत्नी के साथ भी सांझा कर सकते हैं।

इस पत्र की जानकारी को इस्तेमाल करने के लिए आपका स्वागत है परंतु इस बात का ख़ास ख़याल रखें की यदि आपको याददाश्त से सम्बंधित कुछ भी दिक्कतें हो रहीं हैं तो आप कृपया कर डॉक्टर से सलाह करें। कृपया कर इस पत्र को और आपकी भरी हुई पत्रिका को आपके डॉक्टर के पास ले जाएँ। इस पत्र की बातों को आप एक चिकित्सिय सलाह के रूप में ना लें, परंतु इसे अच्छे से पढ़ें और अपना ख्याल रखें। महत्वपूर्ण

याददाश्त से जुड़ी दिक्कतें सामान्य रूप से उम्र बढ़ने से सम्बंधित नहीं होती हैं। अगर आपको वाक़ई में बीमारी हे तो कई तरीक़ें हैं याददाश्त की दिक्कतों से जुड़े लक्षणों को उल्टा करने के, अपने आप को मनोभ्रम से बचाने के और गम्भीर याददाश्त की समस्याओं को रोक के रखने के।

अपना ख़याल रखें एवं स्वस्थ रहें,

तारा

DEAR DAD, CAN WE TALK ABOUT YOUR MEMORY?

## आपकी अभी की याददाश्त की दिक्कतों से सम्बंधित आपके सवाल

प्रिय पिताजी,

आप बता रहे थे कि आपको यादाश्त में दिक्कतें आ रही है, और उससे जुड़े आपके कुछ प्रश्न हैं। मेने सोचा कि पत्र द्वारा आपको सलाह देना सबसे आसान तरीका रहेगा। जैसे की आप जानते हो कि में अल्ज़ाइमर रोग एवं याददाश्त की तकलीफ़ से जुड़े शोध क्षेत्र में कार्यरत हूँ, और इस वजह से में आपको बहुत कुछ बताना चाहती हूँ। आपकी बेटी होने के नाते मुझे लगता है कि यह सलाहें आपके लिए काफ़ी महत्वपूर्ण रहेंगी। इसीलिए आप कृपा कर इसे समझे और ये भी जाने कि यह पत्र में अपने दिल से लिख रही हूँ। यह काफ़ी हद तक शैक्षणिक रूप से केंद्रित है, लेकिन देखा जाए तो ३० साल का अल्ज़ाइमर रोग से जुड़ी खोज का अनुभव इसे शुरुआत करने के लिए सही है।

शुरुआत "याददाश्त की तकलीफ़ों" की जुड़ी हुई बातों से करते हैं। आपने मुझसे पूछा था कि डॉक्टर क्या करेंगे अगर उन्हें पता चलता है कि आपकी याददाश्त के स्तर में दिक्कत है। हो सकता है वे आपसे कहें कि आपको "माइल्ड कोग्निटीव इम्पैरमेंट"(एम सी आइ) (ज्ञान-समबंधि मानसिक हानि) की तकलीफ है। में जानती हूँ कि काफ़ी लोगों को उम्र बढ़ने पर अल्ज़ाइमर रोग या स्मृतिभ्रंश की बीमारी होने का डर रहता है। लेकिन यह पत्र अल्ज़ाइमर रोग या स्मृतिभ्रंश की बीमारी के बारे में नहि है। और सिर्फ़ इसीलिए क्योंकि आपको यादाश्त में दिक्कतें हैं, सीधे किसी निष्कर्ष पर पहुँचना सही नहि होगा। बल्कि, "यादशक्ति में कमी होने की तकलीफ" और "माइल्ड कोग्निटीव इम्पैरमेंट" हकीक़त में क्या हैं, इस विषय पर में आपसे बात करना चाहती हूँ। और इसीलिए यह जाने कि 'एम सी आइ' से जुड़ी नवीनतम खोज पर चिकित्सा क्षेत्र एवं शोधकर्ताओं का फ़िलहाल में क्या कहना है, इस बात की जानकारी हासिल करें, और हो सकता है कि

147

तथ्य जानकर आप थोड़ी राहत महसूस करें जो आपको आगे बढ़ने में मदद कर सकती हैं।

फ़िलहाल हमें जो 'हल्के स्तर की यादशत की तकलीफ़ों' की जानकारी हैं उसके अवलोकन से शुरू करते हैं।

"माइल्ड कोग्निटीव इम्पैरमेंट" यानी आप की यादशक्ति और विचारशक्ति में ध्यान देने योग्य बदलाव होना, जिस तरह के आपने मुझे अपने बारे में बताए थे। लेकिन ये बदलाव जिसमें रोज़मर्रा के कार्यों में मदद की ज़रूरत पड़े इतने ज़्यादा तीव्र या गम्भीर नहीं होते हैं। इस स्तर की यादशत की तकलीफ़ों को "माइल्ड नयूरोकोगनिटिव डिसॉर्डर" (एम एन सी डी) के नाम से भी जाना जाता है, जिसमें ज्ञान समबंधि कामकाज करने में ध्यान देने लायक कमी होती है, और यह कमी उम्र के साथ बढ़ती जाती है। याद रखें: यह स्मृतिभ्रंश की बीमारी या अलज़ाइमर रोग नहि है!

इससे पहले कि में आगे बढ़ूँ, मुझे आपको बताना है के स्मृतिभ्रंश की बीमारी और अलज़ाइमर रोग क्या होते हैं, जिससे कि आपको समझ आ सके कि हम इनमें से किसी भी एक गम्भीर बीमारी की बात नहि कर रहे हैं।

स्मृतिभ्रंश (कभी कभी जिसे बुढ़ापे से होती मानसिक दुर्बलता भी कहा जाता है।) यानी जिसमें आपको नकारी ना जा सकें ऐसी यादाश्त की तकलीफ़ों का अनुभव हो। ठोस रूप से, जिसमें इंसान की विचारने की क्षमता न बचे, यादें याद ना रहें, और ज्ञान समबंधि तर्क ना कर पायें, और तो और रोज़मर्रा के कामों में इस हद तक तकलीफ हो कि इंसान की ज़िंदगी के रोज़ के काम काज करने में असमर्थता होने लग जाए। स्मृतिभ्रंश की तीव्रता, हल्के स्तर से शुरू होते हुए, जिसमें कि शुरुआती तौर पर ज़िंदगी के रोज़ के काम करने में दिक्कतें हों; अति गम्भीर स्थिति पर पहुँचती है जिसमें कि इंसान को हर छोटे से छोटे काम में किसी और की मदद लगने लग जाती है।

अलज़ाइमर रोग स्मृतिभ्रंश की बीमारी होने का एक बड़ा कारण है, पर उसके होने के लिए सिर्फ़ यही एक कारण नहि है। अलज़ाइमर रोग दिमाग़ में दिखने वाली जमी हुई मैल और जालों से चिन्हित किया जाता है। दिमाग़ को घेरे हुई मैल की जमावट प्रोभूजिन (प्रोटीन) तत्वों के जुड़ने से बनी है, और जाले (उलझनें) तब बनती हैं जब महत्वपूर्ण कोशिकाएँ मरने लग जाती हैं और दिमाग़ की ख़ाली जगह को भरती जाती हैं। इसीलिए स्मृतिभ्रंश होने का निदान: यादशक्ति के खोने के गम्भीर लक्षण दिखाई पड़ना और अलज़ाइमर रोग का होना भी एक बड़ा कारण हो सकता है। बहुत सी बीमारियाँ हैं जिससे कि स्मृतिभ्रंश की बीमारी हो सकती है।

**स्मृतिभ्रंश (डिमेंशिया) या अलज़ाइमर रोग का होना, माइल्ड कोग्निटीव इमपैरमेंट (एम सी आइ) से ज़्यादा गम्भीर परिस्थिति है।**

यहाँ पर में आश्वस्त होने की कोशिश कर रही हूँ, में कितना अच्छा कर रही हूँ इस बात से अभी में  असंदिग्ध नहि हूँ।

**<u>यादशक्ति की दिक़्क़तों के स्तर</u>**

| | |
|---|---|
| • **पहला** | **उम्र बढ़ने पर सामान्य स्तर पर यादाश्त की तकलीफ़ें होना** |
| • **दूसरा** | **हल्की गम्भीर यादाश्त की तकलीफ़ जिसे माइल्ड कोग्निटीव इमपैरमेंट (एम सी आइ) कहते हैं।** |
| • **तीसरा** | **अतिशय गम्भीर तकलीफ़ें जिसे स्मृतिभ्रंश (डिमेंशिया) या अलज़ाइमर रोग कहते हैं।** |

That's it.

## रोग-निदान, इलाज, पूर्वानुमान

में बताना चाहूँगी कि हम (रोग-चिकित्सक और शोधकर्ता) रोग को पहचानते हैं, उसके इलाज को जानते हैं, और लम्बे समय तक उस इलाज के असर का अनुमान रखते हैं। आपको जिस तरह की यादाश्त की दिक्क़तें हैं उससे आपको माइल्ड कोग्निटीव इमपैरमेंट होने का अनुमान लगाया जा सकता है।

सब मिलाकर, यह कहा जा सकता है कि १०% से २०% तक ६५ वर्ष या उससे बड़ी उम्र के लोगों को 'एम सी आइ'(MCI) अथवा 'एम एन सी डी'(mNCD) होता है। हम जानते हैं कि इन तकलीफ़ों को होने का जोखिम उम्र के साथ बढ़ता है, और आदमियों में इसका जोखिम औरतों के मुक़ाबले ज़्यादा होता है।

इसीलिए, हालाँकि माइल्ड कोग्निटीव इमपैरमेंट से पीड़ित लोगों में स्मृतिभ्रंश (डिमेंशिया) होने का जोखिम युनाइटेड स्टेट्स में बाक़ियों के मुक़ाबले ज़्यादा है, फिर भी एक बड़ी श्रेणी में जोखिम का आकलन किया जा सकता है (<5% से 20% तक वार्षिक रूपांतरण दरें), लोगों के समूह पर किए गए अध्ययन के अनुसार। अगर किसीमे माइल्ड कोग्निटीव इमपैरमेंट की पहचान होती है, हर एक साल में उस व्यक्ति को डिमेंशिया होने के आसार केवल 5% से कम से लेकर 20% की श्रेणी में होंगे। इसका मतलब कुछ लोगों में सुधार पाया जाता है, कुछ वैसे ही बने रहते हैं, और कुछ की यादाश्त को वाक़ई ज़्यादा हानि पहुँचती है। एक बेटी होने के नाते, में हमेशा यही चाहूँगी के आपकी याद-शक्ति बेहतर होती जाए। बहुत सारी बातें हो सकती हैं जो कि आपकी यादाश्त पर ख़राब असर कर रही हों, इसीलिए चलिए इस पर कुछ कार्यवाही करते हैं ताकि आपकी यादाश्त पहले की तरह सामान्य हो सके।

कई कारण होते हैं जिससे कि वृद्धों में माइल्ड कोग्निटीव इमपैरमेंट या यादशक्ति और

विचारशक्ति में कमी जैसी दिक्क़तें होती हैं, जिसमें की दुखी रहना या तनाव में रहना, कई तरह की दवाइयों का सेवन जो एक दूसरे पर असर कर रही हों, और शरीर में दिल और ख़ून के बहाव से जुड़ी तकलीफ़ें हो सकती है (अनियंत्रित हृदय तथा रक्तवाहिनियों सम्बंधित जोखिम तत्व)। इन चीज़ों पर आपके डॉक्टर तथा स्वास्थय सुविधा प्रदान करने वाले को ध्यान देकर उसपर विचार करने की ज़रूरत है।

इसीलिए पिताजी, अगर आप अभी के हालातों में ख़याल नहि रखेंगे, जब की आपकी यादाश्त ठीक होने के आसार प्रबल हैं, आप हक़ीक़त में कुछ तरह की परिस्थितियों में स्थायी नुकसान कर सकते हैं- इसीलिए कृपया करके आप अपना ख़याल रखें और डॉक्टर से तुरंत जाकर मिलें!


जैसे की आप देख सकते हैं, इस पत्र का सबसे महत्वपूर्ण हिस्सा है कि आप तुरंत डॉक्टर से सम्पर्क करें! और अपना तथा अपनी सेहत का ख़याल रखें। अभी के लिए में आपको बताना चाहती हूँ कि आप किस तरह से अपनी सेहत और यादाश्त से सम्बंधित चीज़ों का ख़याल रखने की शुरुआत कर सकते हैं, एवं  डॉक्टर से मिलने के उपरांत किन बातों को आपके दिमाग़ में रखना है।


## अभी क्या है जो मदद कर सकता है? अपना ख़याल रखें!!

क्या है जो आप के लिए सबसे अधिक सहायक बन सकता है, और यादाश्त की तकलीफ़ों से जुड़े जोखिमों को कम कर सकता है?


सबसे ज़रूरी बात पहले, अपने शरीर तथा दिमाग़ के स्वास्थय का ध्यान रखें। जैसा कि आप जानते ही हैं, यह एक दूसरे से जुड़े हुए हैं। असलियत में अपने आप का ख़याल

रखने से हमारे दिमाग़ के अंदर सकारात्मक शारीरिक परिवर्तन होते हैं। ये सच में बड़ा विस्मयकारी है और कुछ ही सालों पुरानी शोध है। स्वास्थ्यवर्धक आदतें किस तरह से दिमाग़ और उसके कार्यों में सुधारजनक बदलाव लाने में सक्षम हैं, यह काफ़ी सारे नए अनुसंधान (नैदानिक परीक्षण अध्ययनों द्वारा) में देखा जा रहा है। वे असलियत में अनुसंधान के अध्ययन की शुरुआत होने से पहले लोगों के दिमाग़ की बारीकी से जाँच करके उसमें हुए बदलावों को देख सकते हैं तथा उसको नाप सकते हैं, और फिर बीच में नयी हरकतों और आदतों का आचरण करके, जब अध्ययन समाप्त हो जाता है तो वे फिर से लोगों के दिमाग़ को बारीकी से जाँचते हैं। तब शोधकर्ता देख सकते हैं कि किस तरह से डिग से महत्वपूर्ण हिस्सों में वृद्धि हुई है और वो हक़ीक़त में और स्वस्थ हुए हैं। ये इस तरह है जैसे आप व्यायाम करने के बाद या वज़न उठाने के बाद अपने हाथों या पैरों के स्नायुओं को बढ़ता या ज़्यादा ताक़तवर होते देख सकते हैं। यही चीज़ आपके दिमाग़ के लिए भी है। फ़र्क़ इतना है कि हम हमारे दिमाग़ के अंदर होते हुए बदलावों को झाँक के देख नहि सकते, जबतक कि हम किसी तकनीकी इमेजिंग का इस्तेमाल ना करें, जो कि हमें हज़ारों डॉलर की पड़ती है। क्योंकि हमारी याद शक्ति के सुधारने में वक़्त लग सकता है, इन आदतों को छोड़ देना आसान हो जाता है। पर जब हम समय के साथ अपनी यादशक्ति को बेहतर होते देखते हैं, तब इन नयी आदतों को अपनाना और उसे जीवन में उतारना बड़ा ही क़ीमती निर्णय लगता है।

में नीचे दिए गए सारे विषयों पर ज़्यादा नहि लिख रही हूँ क्योंकि उनपर ढेरों किताबें उपलब्ध हैं। में सिर्फ़ आपको ये बताना चाहती हूँ किन मूलभूत क्षेत्रों में काम करके आप स्वस्थ बने रह सकते हैं, जोकि अनुसंधान के अध्ययन में पायी गयी हैं। में जानती हूँ काफ़ी कोशिश लगती है इन चीज़ों को बदलने में और नए कार्यों को ज़िंदगी में शामिल करने में। हालाँकि हम एक ही शहर में नहि हैं, लेकिन तब भी इनमे से कुछ क्षेत्र ऐसे हैं जिनपे में भी काम कर सकती हूँ, तो हो सकता है कभी हम इन्हें साथ में कर पाएँ।

१) **स्वास्थ्यवर्धक खाएँ और पर्याप्त पानी पीएँ।** खाद्य पदार्थ वह खाएँ जो आपके दिल के लिए अच्छे हों। आप "हृदय स्वास्थ्यवर्धक" खाने के बारे में इंटर्नेट पर देख सकते हैं। फल तथा सब्ज़ियाँ, साबुत अनाज, बादाम आदि, बिना चर्बी का मास, एवं मछली। "भूमध्य आहार" के बारे में कहने को बहुत कुछ है। कुछ अध्ययनों में पाया गया है कुछ विटामिन और पोशाक तत्व ऐसे हैं जो कि स्वास्थ्य में सुधार कर सकते हैं। अतः में इसके बारे में आपको ज़्यादा बताउँगी जब अनुसंधान के परिणाम बहार आएँगे। अभी कि लिए, में यह कह सकती हूँ कि ओमेगा-३ बहुत ज़्यादा ज़रूरी है और इसे तैलिय मछली द्वारा प्राप्त करना सबसे अच्छा ज़रिया माना जा सकता है, इनमे चरबियुक्त मछली जैसे कि सैलमन, मैकरल, ओर सार्डिन का समावेश होता है। अभी ऐसे किसी अनुसंधान के बारे में मुझे जानकारी नहि है जो कि जैविक-अजैविक खाद्य पदार्थ की तुलना पर की गई हो, पर क्योंकि आपको थोड़ी बहुत यादशक्ति की दिक्क़तें हैं, मुझे लगता है कि जितना हो सके  आपको जैविक खाद्य पर थोड़ा ज़्यादा ख़र्च करना चाहिए (ऐसा खाना जो किसी भी तरह कि कीटनाशकों या योज्य के इस्तेमाल बिना उगाया गया हो)। आप/हम काफ़ी ख़ुशनसीब हैं कि हम यह ऊपरी ख़र्च को ख़र्च करने में समर्थ हैं। और इसके ऊपर जब आपका दिमाग़ कह रहा है कि उसे सहाय की ज़रूरत है, कृपया करके रासायनिक खाना अपने शरीर में ना डालें जो कि आपके शरीर को तकलीफ़ दे सकता है।

में एक और बात बीच में लाना चाहूँगी जिस्पे कुछ ज़्यादा अनुसंधान नहि किए गए हैं, और वह है एक अच्छे मल्टीविटामिन और आहार को सम्पूर्ण करने वाले पदार्थ का सेवन करें (जिनकी भी आपके प्रदाता आपको सलाह देतें है)। कृपया

करके इन्हें लें। एसा लगता है कि भले ही इस समय पर ज़्यादा खोज नहि की गयी है, लेकिन किसीकी यादाश्त ठीक करने में मदद करने के किए शरीर को सारे लाभ जो उसे मिल सके, उनकी ज़रूरत होती है।

पर्याप्त पानी पीना और जलिकृत रहना बहुत आवश्यक है, क्योंकि निर्जलित होने से कई सारी यादाश्त से जुड़ी तकलीफ़ें हो सकती है।

२) **व्यायाम।** ये मानते हुए कि आपके डॉक्टर के अनुसार आप व्यायाम कर सकते हैं, एक व्यायाम की योजना तैयार कीजिए जिसमें ऐसे कार्यकलाप को शामिल करें जिनसे कि आपकी हृदय गति में बढ़ावा हो, और ऐसे कार्य में शक्ति प्रशिक्षण को श्रेष्ठ माना जाएगा। व्यायाम फ़ायदों के लिए बहुत ही ग़ज़ब का क्षेत्र है, और सबसे अच्छा अनुसंधान भी है जिसमें कि दिमाग़ की इमेजिंग को शामिल किया गया है, जो वास्तविक तौर पे दिमाग़ की संरचना को बदल पाया है, नाकि सिर्फ़ हृदय और माँसपेशियों को।

३) **प्राचुर्य मात्रा में नींद लें।** अगर आप बहुत अच्छी मात्रा में नींद नहि ले रहे हैं, तो अच्छे से सोने के सारे तरीक़ों के बारे में पढ़ें या फिर अपने स्वास्थ्य प्रबंधक से बात करें। मुझे नींद और कचरे की गाड़ी के बीच की समानता बड़ी पसंद है जिसमें कि वर्णन है कि जैसे कचरे की गाड़ी आके कूड़ा-कचरा ले जाती है, उसी तरह नींद सारी गंदगी को आपके दिमाग़ से उठाकर उसे वहाँ से ख़ाली कर देती है। इसीलिए कभी भी नींद को त्याग कर कचरे के निष्कासन को रद्द ना करें। और अब तो ऐसे अनुसंधान अध्ययन भी हैं जो कि यही बात दर्शाते हैं।

४) **अपने दोस्तों और परिवारजनों के साथ समय व्यतीत करें।** सामाजिक बने और दूसरों से बातें करें। लोगों से बातचीत करें। ऐसे अध्ययन हैं जो दर्शाते हैं कि सामाजिक कार्य करना और यादशक्ति कमज़ोर होने में कमी होना, एक दूसरे से जुड़े

हुए हैं। इसका मतलब है कि आपकी यादाश्त लम्बे समय तक अच्छी बनी रहेगी। शोधकर्ताओं ने दर्शाया है कि वो लोग जो दूसरे लोगों के सम्पर्क में ज़्यादा आते हैं, वह यादशक्ति से जुड़े परीक्षण में ज़्यादा अच्छा करते हैं।

**५) जोखिम कम करने में संलग्न होना।** जोखिम कम करना यानी वो चीज़ें करना बंद करना जो कि हम जानते हैं कि हमारे शरीर और हृदय कि लिए सही नहि है। धूम्रपान इसका एक अच्छा उदाहरण है। हम जानते हैं कि यह हमारे सम्पूर्ण स्वास्थ्य के लिए ख़राब है, और यह वास्तविक रूप से हमारे दिमाग़ पर भी असर करता है।

एक स्वस्थ हृदय बहुत ज़रूरी है हमारे दिमाग़ के लिए। यह बोध की बात है। हमें चाहिए कि ख़ून दिल से दिमाग़ तक जाए, इसीलिए हमें एक स्वस्थ हृदय की ज़रूरत है। और ख़ून ही ग्लूकोज़ या रकतशर्करा  को दिमाग़ तक ले जाता है। और इसीलिए या दिमाग़ के लिए शक्ति होती है। तो, अगर किसिको ग़लत रकतशर्करा  है और यह उनके दिमाग़ में जा रहा है, थोड़ा ज़्यादा थोड़ा काम या पूरी जगह पर तो वह दिमाग़ में तबाही मचा सकता है और याददाश्त की तकलीफ़ें पैदा कर सकता है।

**क) धूम्रपान बंद करें।** अगर आप फिरसे धूम्रपान कर रहे हैं, तो कृपया करके रुक जाएँ। और तो और ऐसे किसी के आसपास भी ना रहें जो धूम्रपान करता हो, क्योंकि सेकंड हैंड स्मोकिंग भी नुकसानकारी है।

**ख) मधुमेह।** क्या आपने आपकी रकतशर्करा की जाँच करवायी है? क्योंकि अब हम ये जानते हैं है कि मधुमेह, और यहाँ तक कि मधुमेह होने से पहले का स्तर (जब रकतशर्करा का स्तर ऊपर-नीचे  जा रहा हो, और नियमित ना रहे पा रहा हो) डिमेंशिया से जुड़ा हुआ है। कृपया कर चीनी के वपराश को भी बंद करें।

**ग) उच्च रक्तचाप या अतिरक्तदाब।** अपने रक्तचाप को नियंत्रित रखना बहुत ज़रूरी है। ज़रा उसके बारे में सोचिए- दिमाग़ पर ज़रूरत से ज़्यादा दबाव होना, हमारे लिए अच्छा नहि है।

**घ) तनाव और चिंता।** अनुसंधान दर्शाते हैं कि वह लोग जिन्हें तनाव और चिंता रहते हैं, उन्हें यादाश्त से जुड़ी तकलीफ़ें ज़्यादा होने की सम्भावना रहती है। पक्की तरीक़े से नहि कहा जा सकता कि ऐसा क्यों है, लेकिन इससे मतलब यह है कि इन भावनाओं का इलाज करें और मदद लें। इससे जुड़े बहुत सारे इलाज उपलब्ध हैं अगर आप इन्हें अभी अनुभव कर रहे हो तो।

**च) शोध।** शरीर में शोध का होना हमारे लिए अच्छा नहि है। शरीर के हिस्से का भाग जहाँ पे सिर गर्दन पर बैठता है (जिसे रुधिर मस्तिष्क रोध कहा जाता है) उस पर शोध का होना विशेष रूप से बुरा है। अगर रुधिर मस्तिष्क रोध (ब्लड ब्रेन बैरीअर) के छोटे से मार्ग में जहाँ से रीड़ द्रव्य दिमाग़ की और जाता है, उसपर सूजन है, तो वह थोड़ा और खूल जाएगा और इसका मतलब होगा कि दूसरी चीज़ें भी दिमाग़ की और बढ़ेंगी और फिर वे वहाँ उत्पात मचा देंगी। इसका मतलब है अपने शरीर का ख़याल रखना, जिसमें दाँत चिकित्सक के पास जाना भी शामिल है जिससे कि आपको मसूड़ों की बीमारी ना हो पाए (जोकि शरीर में एक प्रकार का शोध है)।

**६) दिमाग़ का उपयोग।** यह सच है कि जिस तरह से शरीर को व्यायाम की ज़रूरत होती है, उसी तरह हमारे दिमाग़ को भी उपयोगिता की ज़रूरत होती है। अपने दिमाग़ को मानसिक रूप से चुनौतिपूर्ण गतिविधियों से जोड़ें। ये कुछ भी हो सकता है जो कि आपको अच्छा लगता हो। खेल खेलना, पहलियाँ सुलझाना, पढ़ना, नई चीज़ें सिखना, किसी तरीक़े का शौक़ होना। ये स्वैच्छा से दूसरों की मदद करना भी हो सकता है, ख़ास करके सेवनिवृति के साथ।

**७) तनाव कम करें।** लम्बे समय तक तनाव में रहना वास्तविक रूप से दिमाग़ को नुकसान पहुँचा सकता है, जिससे सिखना और भी मुश्किल बन सकता है और यह यादशक्ति की तकलीफ़ें भी उत्पन्न करता है। ध्यान में बैठना, योग, और इस तरह की दिमाग़-शरीर से जुड़े कार्य, इन तरह की तकलीफ़ों में काफ़ी सुधार लाते नज़र आए हैं। ध्यान में बैठने से और योग से काफ़ी अच्छा सुधार देखा गया है इस तरीक़े की कई दिक्कतों में। यहाँ तक कि ध्यान और योग हमारे दिमाग़ की संरचना में ऐसे बदलाव लाते हैं जिससे शोध यादाश्त के क्षेत्रों से कम होता पाया जा सकता है।

**८) संगीत।** क्योंकि आपको संगीत बड़ा प्रिय है, आप अपने पसंदिता गानें और धुन सुना कीजिए। मुझे लगता है यह आपको ज़्यादा ख़ुश करेगा। और तो और एक नया अनुसंधान है जो दर्शाता है कि कैसे संगीत दिमाग़ के अलग अलग हिस्सों को प्रोत्साहित करता है।

**९) प्रेम करें और कृतज्ञता रखें।** प्रार्थना करें और आभारी रहें। आप ने मुझे मेरी ज़िंदगी में ये सिखाया है, तो क्या अब में ही आपको ये बात कह सकती हूँ? यहाँ में ध्यान में बैठना, और भगवान कि साथ विलीन होना भी शामिल कर सकती हूँ, लेकिन आप वो पहले ही करते हो। में अपनी इस आख़री अंक में दी गयी सलाह के अनुसंधान को लेकर निश्चिन्त नहि हूँ, पर में इससे ज़्यादा बेहतर सलाह के बारे में नहि सोच सकती हूँ।

दिमाग़ के स्वास्थ्य सम्बंधित ये काफ़ी सारे सुझाव हैं। अभी के लिए आपको जो सही लगे, आप उसे चुन लें।

### डॉक्टर या स्वास्थ्य प्रबंधक से मिलना

ठीक है, अब बात करते हैं डॉक्टर या स्वास्थ्य प्रबंधक के पास जाकर अपनी याददाश्त की तकलीफ़ों की जाँच कराने की। यह बहुत ज़रूरी है। में इस विषय पर थोड़ी तकनीकी होने जा रही हूँ, लेकिन क्योंकि हम दोनो अस्पताल में काम कर चुके हैं, मुझे लगता है आप पास पहले से काफ़ी सारी जानकारियाँ होंगी जो कि आपके काम आ सकती हैं।

157

अगर आप मेरे पक्ष से निश्चिन्त नहि हो, तो कृपया करके अपने डॉक्टर से कहना कि वो आपको इस बारे में विस्तार से समझा सके।

## नियोग के लिए

डॉक्टर से मिलने के समय पर किसिको अपने साथ अवश्य ले जाएँ।

यह एक महत्वपूर्ण सलाह है। अगर आप अपने किसी क़रीबी को साथ लेकर जाएँगे तो ये आपको काफ़ी मददगार साबित होगा, किसी ऐसे को जिससे आप काफ़ी अच्छे से जानते हों (जैसे की माँ), जो आपकी यादाश्त से जुड़ी तकलीफ़ों की पुष्टि कर सके और डॉक्टर तक यह संदेश पहुँचा सके कि आप चाहते हैं कि डॉक्टर आपकी इस तकलीफ़ को गम्भीरता से ले। माँ (या जिसे भी आप साथ ले जाएँ) छोटी छोटी बातों को लिख सकती हैं, जब आप सिर्फ़ डॉक्टर को अच्छे से सुन रहे हों।

डॉक्टर को क्या जाँचने की ज़रूरत है अगर आपको यादाश्त में दिक्कत है या 'एम सी आइ' है?

डॉक्टर को आपकी ज़िंदगी के इन पहलुओं को समझने की ज़रूरत है: (आप इसमें मदद के तौर पर लिखके नोट्स बना सकते हो और इस सूची को डॉक्टर से मिलने के निस्चित समय पर साथ ले जा सकते हो)।

१) यादाश्त/ ज्ञान समबंधि कार्यों में बदलाव। (बदलाव कब शुरू हुए, कैसे हुए, यादाश्त की दिक़्क़तों  के कुछ उदाहरण)

२) रोजर्मरा के काम करने की क्षमता में बदलाव। इसमें दैनिक जीविका के कार्य, या आप किस तरह आप का दिन बिताते हैं, और आपको क्या तकलीफ़ें रहती हैं जब आप वित्त सम्बंधित कार्य करते हैं।

३) क्या आप अच्छे से खा रहे हैं, और आपके पीने के बारे में क्या कहेंगे? हाँ जी, दोनो पानी और शराब! याद रखें कि निर्जलित होना (पर्याप्त पानी ना पीना) भी यादाश्त की तकलीफ़ें करने में समर्थ है।

४) अभी के दवाई के पर्चे और बिना पर्ची की दवाइयाँ। इसमें विटामिन और आहार का पोषण सम्पूर्ण करने के पदार्थ भी शामिल हैं।

५) दिमाग़ से जुड़े हुए लक्षण जैसे कि: सुनना, देखना, बोलना, नींद की तकलीफ़ें, चलना, सून्न पड़ना, या शरीर के किसी भी हिस्से में झुनझुनी होना।

६) हृदय से जुड़े हुए लक्षण- मतलब कि जब दिमाग़ को हृदय द्वारा सही मात्रा में पर्याप्त ख़ून मिलता है, तो उसे सही मात्रा में ग्लूकोज़/रक्तशर्करा भी मिल जाती है। मैंने पहले भी इसका उल्लेख किया था। इसीलिए अगर आपको उच्च रक्तचाप के कोई भी लक्षण हैं, मधुमेह से पहले का स्तर, या मधुमेह है, या किसी भी तरह की हृदय की बीमारी है जैसे कि असामान्य दिल की गति, तो आप तैयार रहें अपने चिकित्सक से विचार-विमश करने कि लिए।

७) दिमाग़ी स्वास्थ्य या सलामती की तकलीफ़ें जैसे की तनाव या चिंता से व्यवहार या व्यक्तित्व में परिवर्तन आना, ये भी कारण हो सकते हैं यादाश्त की तकलीफ़ों के।

८) परिवार का इतिहास। डॉक्टर आपके परिवार के इतिहास के बारे में भी जानना चाहेगा। जहाँ तक मुझे पता है, खुशनसीबी से हमारे परिवार में किसिको गम्भीर यादाश्त खोने की बीमारी या डिमेंशिया नहि रहा है। लेकिन, पापा, अगर आपको ऐसा कुछ परिवार के बारे में पता है, तो डॉक्टर को अवश्य बताएँ।

स्वास्थ्य चिकित्सक या प्रभंधक कुछ शारीरिक जाँच और साथ ही तंत्रिकाओं से सम्बंधित जाँचे करना चाहेगा। में चाहती हूँ कि डॉक्टर के पास आपसे प्रश्न पूछने का मौक़ा हो, और आप की शारीरिक जाँच भी करे, ताकि हम समझ पाएँ कि आखिर चल क्या रहा है।

## प्रयोगशाला में किए जाने वाली ख़ून की जाँच

प्रयोगशाला के काम या वहाँ पे की जाने वाली जाँच के बारे में पूछें कि क्या ये आपकी उम्र के अनुसार सामान्य है, क्योंकि आपकी यादशक्ति को लेकर की चिंता किसी विटामिन या मिनरल की कमी की वजह से भी हो, जोकि आपकी यादशक्ति को कमज़ोर कर रही हो।

ये कुछ है जो में जानती हूँ कि आप को परीक्षण करने के लिए कहना चाहिए, कम से कम जब आपके पास स्वास्थ्य बीमा है। ख़ून की जाँच सम्पूर्ण उपापचयी सूची को शामिल करती है, यह सब शामिल करना ज़रूरी है: सम्पूर्ण रक्त जाँच, इलेक्ट्रोलाइट्स, ग्लूकोज़, केलशियम, अवटुग्रंथि का कार्य, आइरन, विटामिन बी१२, और फोलेट। पर आपके डॉक्टर को आपके ख़ून के और भी हिस्सों के कामकाज को जाँचना हो सकता है।

आप ये सारी जाँच आपके ख़ून पर करवाना चाहें इसके पीछे कारण है कि आप जितना हो सके 'एम सी आइ'(MCI) होने के लिए जुड़े कारण की जड़ को पहचान कर उसे पहले की तरह सामान्य कर सकें। इनमे जैसे की रोगसंक्रमण, गुर्दे की समस्याएँ, बहुत कम या बहुत ज़्यादा मेगनेशियम, बहुत कम या बहुत ज़्यादा केलशियम, रक्तशर्करा/ शर्करा के स्तर की तकलीफ़ें (मधुमेह), अवटुग्रंथि से जुड़ी तकलीफ़ें, विटामिन या पोशाक तत्वों से दिक्क़तें (जैसे की विटामिन बी१२, आइरन, फोलेट की कमी)। ये कोई आश्चर्य की बात नहि होगी कि आपको दिए गए अमेरिकन आहार की वजह से इनही में से कुछ आपको निकल आए। (आपके लिए यह एक बुरा मज़ाक़ था)

अतिरिक्त प्रयोगशाला की जाँच, गुर्दे के कार्य और जिगर के कार्यों को परखने के लिए की जा सकती है। और लाइम नामक बीमारी, सिफ़िलस, और एच आइ वी, ज्ञान समबंधि हानि से जुड़े असामान्य कारण ज़ाहिर कर सकते हैं।

नींद से जुड़े श्वासरोध के लिए भी प्रयोगशाला परीक्षण उपलब्ध है। अगर कभी आप खराटे लेते हो या आपको रात में सामान्य तरीक़े से साँस लेने में दिक़्क़त आती हो, तो

160

ये आपके ध्यान केंद्रित करने की शक्ति को प्रभावित कर सकती है, और दिन के दौरान यादाश्त को भी प्रभावित कर सकती है।

## वृतिक का दवाइयों के प्रति गुण दोष निरूपण: क्यों?

आपको चाहिए कि आप किसी वृतिक से आपकी दवाइयों के गुण एवं दोषों का निरूपण करें। आपको यह पता है क्योंकि आप एक फ़ार्मासिस्ट रह चुके हो, और यह यादाश्त से जुड़ी तकलीफ़ों वाले लोगों के लिए बहुत ज़रूरी है। कुछ दवाइयों के दर्जे और मिश्रण भी एक कारण हो सकते हैं यादाश्त की तकलीफ़ होने के, इसीलिए अभी के सारी दवाइयों के पर्चे, बिना पर्चे की दवाइयाँ, विटामिन, इन सब पर पुनर्विचार करना चाहिए।

फ़िलहाल आपको ये जानने की बिलकुल आवश्यकता नहि है, लेकिन दवाइयों के दर्जों के प्रकार ज्ञान शक्ति से सम्बंधित बीमारियों के कारण हों, ये बड़ा ही लाज़मी है। दवाइयों के क्लास जैसे की ऐनटीकोलिनर्जिक, ओपीएटस निंद्राकर औषध, बेनज़ोड़ाएजापिंस, नोन बेनज़ोड़ाएजापिन हिप्नोटिक्स (निंद्राजनक) (उदाहरण: जोल्पीडेम), डिगोक्सिन, एंटीहिस्टेमाइंस, ट्रीसाइक्लिक एंटीडिपरेसनट्स , स्केलेटल मसल रिलेक्संट, और एंटीएपीलेपटिक्स। रजोनिवृति में काम आते होर्मोन सम्बंधित इलाज (सिर्फ़ इस्ट्रोजन या इस्ट्रोजन के साथ प्रोजेस्टिन) से पाया गया है कि ये 'एम सी आइ'(MCI) या डिमेंशिया (स्मृतिभ्रंश) होने का जोखिम बढ़ाती हैं। (ऐसा नहि है कि ये आपपे लागू होता है। ये बस आपकी जानकारी कि लिए था, हो सकता है ये बात आपको मज़ेदार लगे।)। इसके उपरांत, उच्च रक्तचाप में दी जाने वाली दाबहासी दवाएँ, फिर रक्तशर्करा की तकलीफ़ों से जुड़ी दिक्कतों जैसे की रक्तशर्करा कम होना, रक्तशर्करा बढ़ी होना, मधुमेह से पहले का स्तर, और मधुमेह भी ज्ञान शक्ति से सम्बंधित तकलीफ़ों का कारण हो सकती है।

## यादाश्त या ज्ञान समबंधि परीक्षण

हम चाहते हैं को कोई आपका यादाश्त या ज्ञान समबंधि परीक्षण करे। एक स्वास्थ्य सम्भाल वृत्तिक भी बड़े ही सामान्य सा यादाश्त या ज्ञान समबंधि परीक्षण करते हैं, जिसके लिए १० से २० मिनट लगते हैं। एसे कई तरह के अलग परीक्षण होते हैं जो एक चिकित्सक उपयोग में लेते है, और हो सकता है कि वे 'मोनट्रीआल कॉग्निटिव असेस्मेंट' नामक परीक्षण, मिनी कॉग्निटिव औज़ार, या मेरा मनपसंद, ३एमएस ( मोडिफ़ाइड मिनी मेंटल स्टेट) का परीक्षण। अगर चिकित्सक इससे ज़्यादा परीक्षण करना चाहे, तो बस ख़ुश होना के आप पर और भी अच्छा और विकसित परीक्षण हो रहा है। इसके परिणाम बड़े ही सहायक साबित होंगे। और अगर डॉक्टर फिरसे ६ महीने या साल भर बाद आपसे बात करें, तब आप समझ पाएँगे कि यादाश्त में बदलाव हुआ है, या हाल वैसा ही है। आपका सबसे पहला यादाश्त से जुड़े टेस्ट को 'बेसलाइन' कहा गया है, और फिरसे, इससे कराना बड़ा ही सहायक रहेगा।

## दिमाग़ की बारीकी जाँच के लिए कहना: दिमाग़ का तकनीकी प्रतिबिम्ब बनवाना।

आज की प्रौध्योगिकी (टेकनोलजी) बढ़ी ही ग़ज़ब की है, और अगर ऐसा लगे कि आपको यादाश्त में तकलीफ़ हो रही है, तो हो सकता है आपके डॉक्टर आपके दिमाग़ की बारीकी से जाँच करवाएँ- या आपके दिमाग़ के प्रतिबिंब (इमेज) बनवाएँ। कृपया कर आप इस बात पे अपनी सहमति देना। यह बिलकुल ही पिडरहित है, आपको बस ३०-४५ मिनट के लिए एक यंत्र (मशीन) में लेटना रहेगा, और इससे वे आपके दिमाग़ की तस्वीरें ले पाएँगे।

कुछ दो तीन अलग परीक्षण होते हैं जो आपके दिमाग़ की तस्वीरें निकालने में समर्थ हैं। एक है मैग्नेटिक रेज़ोनेंस इमेजिंग (MRI) या CT स्कैन (कम्प्यूटरायज़्ड टोमोग्राफ़ी, साथ

ही कहा जाता है CAT स्कैन जिसे कम्प्यूटरायज्ड ऐक्सीयल टोमोग्राफी) दोनो ही अच्छे परीक्षण हैं। सामान्य तौर पर डॉक्टर इनमे से सिर्फ़ एक ही करवाने को कहते हैं।

आख़िर वे इन तरह दिमाग़ी जाँच क्यों करते हैं? यह देखने के लिए कि दिमाग़ में कहीं कोई गिठान, रक्तस्त्राव या रोग संक्रमण तो नहि है। और क्योंकि हम सभी के दिमाग़ सिकुड़ते हैं, डॉक्टर "सार्वत्रिक घन विस्तार" (ग्लोबल मास वॉल्यूम) पर भी नज़र डालते हैं, यह देखने के लिए कि उम्र के अनुसार ही आप का दिमाग़ सिकुड़ रहा है या नहि, कहीं उससे बढ़कर सिकुड़न तो नज़र नहि आ रही है। वे और भी तरह के दिमाग़ में होते संरचनात्मक बदलावों पर नज़ार डालते हैं, यह देखने के लिए कहीं कुछ असाधारण तो नहि है।

ये और इस तरह के दूसरे परीक्षण एक मूलभूत "बेसलाइन" तौर पे करना अच्छा होता है, जैसे की में पहले भी कह चुकी हूँ। और अगर आपको अभी भी यादाश्त की तकलीफ़ें रहती हैं, इन एक से दो सालों में, जो कि खुदसे ठीक नहि हो पाती हैं, तब डॉक्टर दूसरी जाँच "स्कैन" करवा सकते हैं, और फिर दोनो में तुलना कर सकते हैं।

तकनीकी प्रतिबिम्ब बनवाने (इमेजिंग) का एक और फ़ायदा यह है कि अगर आपको कभी भी स्ट्रोक आया हो, एक शांत स्ट्रोक ही सही (मतलब जिसकी आपको जानकारी ना हो।) या क्षणिक स्थानिक-अरक्तता संबंधी हमला (ट्रानसिएन्ट इश्चेमिक अटेक) हुआ हो, तो हो सकता है उस वजह से आपकी यादाश्त खोयी हो, पर थोड़ी बहुत या सारी ही वापिस भी आ गयी हो। काफ़ी बार इस तरह कि स्ट्रोक दिमाग़ी जाँच के दौरान देखने में आ जाते हैं, और यह बहुत ज़रूरी है, क्योंकि इसके बाद आप एक हृदय रोग विशेषज्ञ या मस्तिष्क रोग विशेषज्ञ से मिलना चाहेंगे, जिससे की आप इन स्वास्थ्य समबंधि तकलीफ़ों को काम कर पाएँ या रोक पाएँ- और पक्का कर पाएँ कि ये दोबारा से ना हों!

163

## हमें इस मूल्याँकन और परिक्षणो के परिणामों से क्या मिलता है?

अगर इनमे से कोई भी परिणाम या उपादान महत्वपूर्ण निकलते हैं, तो फिर डॉक्टर उन लक्षणो को ठीक करने की कोशिश करता है, यह देखने के लिए कि क्या इससे आपकी यादाश्त ठीक होने में मदद मिल पाती है या नहि। चिकित्सक आपसे और आपके परिवार कि लोगों से (जो भी आपके साथ नियुक्ति कि समय पर साथ गए थे) MCI के निदान दौरान क्या पाया गया था इसपे भी चर्चा कर सकता है।

दोनो ही बातों में, चिकित्सक आपको छः महीनो में फिरसे मिलना चाहेगा। इसीलिए, हर छः महीनो में  फिरसे मिलने का समय निश्चीत करना महत्वपूर्ण है, जिससे कि डॉक्टर आपके अंदर यादाश्त/ ज्ञान समबंधि एवं ज़रूरतों के बदलावों को देख सके (चाहे फिर वो सुधार के लक्षण ही हों)।

## कृपया कर ज़रूरत लगने पर परामर्श करें।

अगर आपको यादाश्त से जुड़ी गम्भीर तकलीफ़ें हैं, में चाहूँगी के आपके प्राथमिक देखभाल चिकित्सक आपको किसी विशेषज्ञ के पास भेजें। क्योंकि विशेषज्ञ की सलाह महत्वपूर्ण है और वे समझते हैं कौनसी जाँचे करवाना ज़रूरी है, और आपके लिए क्या मददगार साबित हो सकता है। यह कोई मस्तिष्क रोग विशेषज्ञ या जराचिकित्सा विशेषज्ञ (कोई ऐसा जो वृद्धों के लिए काम करता हो) हो सकता है।

## "माइल्ड कोग्निटीव इमपैरमेंट"(एम सी आइ) (ज्ञान-समबंधि मानसिक हानि) की परख

## "माइल्ड कोग्निटीव इमपैरमेंट"(एम सी आइ) को परखने के लिए कौनसी जानकारी ज़रूरी है।

यह कुछ जानकारियाँ हैं जो डॉक्टर "माइल्ड कोग्निटीव इमपैरमेंट"(एम सी आइ) को परखने में इस्तेमाल कर सकता है, लेकिन ध्यान दें कि यह निकश कभी भी बदल सकते हैं:

१) इंसान की विचार करने की क्षमताओं में बदलाव पर चिंता के विषय पर खुद उस इंसान से, या उसके किसी जानने वाले से, या फिर चिकित्सक से जिसने उसका निरीक्षण किया हो।

२) एक या उससे अधिक ज्ञान समबंधि क्षेत्र में ख़राबी के "विषयनिष्ट सबूत" (ऊपर परीक्षण में देखें), जिसमें यादाश्त, कार्यकारी काम, ध्यान, भाषा, और स्थानिक-दृष्टि के कौशल।

३) स्वतंत्र रूप से कार्य करने में सक्षम रखने की कोशिश करना (हो सकता है इंसान थोड़ा कम कुशल हो और रोजर्मरा के ज़रूरी काम करने में पहले के मुक़ाबले ज़्यादा भूल करे)

४) सामाजिक या व्यवसायिक कार्य करने में क्षति होने का कोई सबूत ना हो। (यानी डिमेंशिया की तकलीफ़ ना हो)

में उम्मीद करती हूँ कि आप देख सकते हो कि यह सूची कुछ तकलीफ़ें दर्शा रही है, जो ज़्यादा गम्भीर तकलीफ़ें नहि है, और इनही को अभी "माइल्ड कोग्निटीव इमपैरमेंट"(एम सी आइ) की तकलीफ़ के  वर्गीकरण में शामिल किया गया है।

यह ही इसका विवरण है और जो प्राथमिक देखबाल प्रदाता या चिकित्सक आपको मदद करने के लिए  कर सकते हैं। अब में आपसे कुछ और बातों के बारे में बात करना चाहती हूँ, जो कि आप डॉक्टर कि दवाखाने से बहार निकलने के बाद कर सकते हैं, जो कि आपकी यादशक्ति को सबल रखने में आपकी मदद करेंगी।

कृपया करके आप अपने प्राथमिक सम्भाल चिकित्सक/सामान्य चिकित्सक से मिलने के लिए समय नियुक्त करें, और अगर आप चाहें तो, नीचे दिए गए १०-सप्ताह पत्रिका एवं कार्यपत्रकों का खुदसे इस्तेमाल करें और इन्हें आपके चिकित्सक के पास ले जाया करें। आप यह पत्रिका और कार्यपत्र खुदसे भर सकते हैं, लेकिन कभी कभी आपके करीबी लोग इसे भरने के लिए ज़्यादा उपयुक्त होतें हैं। चाहें तो माँ आपके लिए इसे भर सकतीं हैं, या हम इसे फ़ोन पर साथ में भर सकते हैं। आप को जैसा सही लगे, आप मुझे बताइएगा।

उम्मीद करती हूँ आपको यह पत्र सहायक लग रहा है। में समझ सकती हूँ कि यह एक लम्बा पत्र है, लेकिन में चाहती थी कि आपको इन बातों की जानकारी हो क्योंकि यह मेरे ही काम का क्षेत्र है। में आपके साथ हमेशा हूँ, कृपया कर कभी भी कॉल करें।

पापा, में आपसे बहुत प्यार करती हूँ। आप हमेशा मेरी प्रार्थनाओं में रहते हो। भगवान से यही प्रार्थना है कि वे आपको अच्छी सेहत और स्वास्थ्य एवं शांति प्रदान करें।

ढेर सारा प्यार,

तारा रोज़

# Am I Having Memory Problems or Is This Normal?
# क्या मुझे यादाश्त की बीमारी है या ये सामान्य है?
## Worksheet कार्यपत्रक

अपने स्वास्थ्य देखभाल प्रदाता के कार्यालय में जाने से पहले इस प्रपत्र को भरें- और इसे मिलने कि समय पर अपने साथ लेकर आएँ। चिकित्सकों के पास ज़्यादा वक़्त नहि रहता है, पहले के ज़माने की तरह तो बिलकुल भी नहीं, इसीलिए इसे पहले से भर कर मिलने के समय साथ ले जाना फ़ायदेकारक रहेगा, और बाद में जब उनसे मिलने का समय समाप्त हो रहा हो तब इसे डॉक्टर को दिखा सकते हैं

Your name: आपका नाम_____

Doctor/Health Care Provider: डॉक्टर/ स्वास्थ्य सम्भाल प्रदाता

_____

Appointment. Date: नियुक्ति की तारीख़_____

Doctor's/Provider's Phone Number: डॉक्टर/प्रदाता का संपर्क नंबर

_____

I have concerns about my memory. I've written some notes and filled out this form about my memory concerns. Would you like me to read my notes? You can make a copy if you like.

मुझे मेरी यादाश्त को लेकर चिंताएँ हैं। मेरी यादाश्त की तकलीफ़ के बारे में मेने कुछ नोट्स लिखें हैं और इस प्रपत्र को भरा है। क्या आप चाहते हैं कि में इन्हें आपको पढ़कर सुनाऊँ? आप चाहें तो इसकी एक कॉपी बनाकर रख सकते हैं।

MEMORY: I am concerned about these things and I would like to know if this is normal or not: याददाश्त: मुझे इन बातों की चिंता है और में जानना चाहता/चाहती हूँ कि क्या ये सामान्य है या नहि?

_____

I am concerned about my memory, when I: मुझे मेरी याददाश्त की चिंता होती है, जब में: ______________________________

I am also concerned about my memory, when I मुझे मेरी याददाश्त की चिंता तब भी होती है, जब में: ______________________________

Another memory concern I have is: दूसरी याददाश्त से जुड़ी चिंता जो मुझे है, वो यह है कि: ______________________

Does anything make the memory problems worse or better? Are the memory concerns all the time or just sometimes (and when)?
क्या कुछ ऐसा है जो याददाश्त कि दिक़्क़त में सुधार या ख़राबी करता है? क्या याददाश्त से जुड़ी तकलीफ़ पूरे समय रहती है या फिर सिर्फ़ कभी-कबार (और किस वक़्त पे)?

1. ______________________________
2. ______________________________

These memory concern affect my day-to-day life by:
ये याददाश्त की तकलीफ़ मेरी रोजमर्रा की ज़िंदगी को इस तरह से प्रभावित कर रहीं हैं:

1. ______________________________
2. ______________________________

**Medications, other physical problems**: दवाइयाँ, दुसरी शारीरिक तकलीफ़ें:

______________________________

Mental health or well-being problems: मानसिक स्वास्थ्य या सलामती से जुड़ी तकलीफ़ें: ☐ Anxious or Anxiety बेचैनी या व्याकुलता

☐ Sadness or Depression उदासी या अवसाद

______________________________

Other problems in your life (short list) (changes or things/events that are stressful or not easy to deal with): आपकी ज़िंदगी की दुसरी तकलीफ़ें (एक छोटी सूची) (कुछ चीज़ों/मौक़ों पर हुए बदलाव जो तनावपूर्ण हों या आसानी से सूलझाने लायक ना हों: ______________________________

______________________

**Here are some things you may want to say to your doctor/health care professional at your appointment:**

ये कुछ बातें हैं जो हो सकता है आप अपने डॉक्टर/ स्वास्थ्य सम्भाल विशेषज्ञ को उनसे मिलने के समय पर कहना चाहते हों।

"Can you do a memory screening test for me? Either at this appointment or at another appointment? I hear it only takes 10-15 minutes and I would like to know if there is a possible problem."

"क्या आप मेरी एक स्मृति सम्बंधित जाँच या परीक्षण कर सकते हैं? इस नियुक्ति के दौरान या अगली बार जब मिलना निश्चित हो तब? मेने सुना है इसमें केवल १०-१५ मिनट ही लगते हैं और में जानना चाहूँगा अगर वाक़ई में कोई तकलीफ़ हो?"

"If it seems there might be a problem or a possible question about my memory, I would like some blood work to be done to make sure I don't have any causes of memory problems that are reversible, like a vitamin deficiency. Here is a letter my daughter wrote that lists the kinds of blood work that I may need."

"अगर ऐसा लगता है कि मेरी याददाश्त को लेकर कोई परेशानी या कोई प्रश्न हो सकता है, में ख़ून की जाँच के द्वारा निश्चित करना चाहूँगा कि मेरी इस याददाश्त की तकलीफ़ के लिए कोई ऐसा कारण तो ज़िम्मेदार नहि है जिसे फिरसे ठीक किया जा सकता हो, जैसे कि विटामिन की कमी। यह एक पत्र है जो मेरी बेटी ने लिखा है, जिसमें उसने इस तकलीफ़ से जुड़ी सारी ख़ून की जाँचो की सूची बनायी है जिनकी मुझे ज़रूरत लग सकती है।"

Can you also check my medications to make sure there aren't any interactions?"

क्या आप मेरी दवाइयाँ भी जाँच सकते हैं, यह पक्का करने के लिए कि इनका आपस में किसी प्रकार का पारस्परिक प्रभाव तो नहि है?

---

# DEAR DAD, CAN WE TALK ABOUT YOUR MEMORY?

# Am I Having Memory Problems

# क्या मुझे याददाश्त की तकलीफ़ें हैं
## A 10-Week Journal
## १०-साप्ताहिक पत्रिका

Week [सप्ताह]: ☐ 1  ☐ 2  ☐ 3  ☐ 4  ☐ 5  ☐ 6  ☐ 7  ☐ 8  ☐ 9  ☐ 10

Today's date is [आज की तारीख़ है]:

_____

☐ Monday [सोमवार]  ☐ Tuesday [मंगलवार]  ☐ Wednesday [बुधवार]
☐ Thursday[गुरुवार]  ☐ Friday [शुक्रवार]  ☐ Saturday [शनिवार]
☐ Sunday [रविवार]

Big and small activities of the week or day: [सप्ताह या दिन के बड़े और छोटे कार्य]:

_____

## Keeping Track of What I Am Forgetting
## [में क्या भूल रहा/रही हूँ उसपे ध्यान देना]

**My Memory issues/Forgetfulness this week:**
**[मेरी याददाश्त की तकलीफ़/ इस हफ़्ते में हुई विस्मृति]:**
Did I forget something or have concerns about my memory today?
[क्या में कुछ भूला/भूली या आज मुझे याद रखने में कोई तकलीफ़ हुई?]
☐ Yes [हाँ]  ☐ No [ना]  ☐ Maybe [हो सकता है]

**This week, did I forget or have trouble with:** *(check if you had problems)*

_____

**इस हफ़्ते, क्या में भूला या मुझे भूलने सम्बंधित तकलीफ़ हुई:** *(अगर आपको तकलीफ़ हैं तो उसपर ध्यान दें).*

## Forgetfulness विस्मृति:

☐ Names नाम ☐ Keys चाबियाँ      ☐ Wallet/bag/money बँटवा/बेग/रुपए

☐ Cell phone मोबाइल फ़ोन ☐ What I wanted to say जो मुझे कहना था

☐ Something else important कुछ और ज़रूरी बात _____

## Location स्थान:

☐ Forgot day of the week हफ़्ते का दिन भूलना

☐ Forgot where I was में जहाँ था वह स्थान को भूलना

## Felt confused उलझन महसूस होना]:

☐ What was I about to do [में क्या करने वाला था

☐ How to do something I normally do में सामन्यता जो करता हूँ, उसे कैसे करूँ

## Lost खोया हुआ:

☐ Couldn't remember how to get somewhere कहीं कैसे पहुँचना है ये याद न कर पाना

## Basics मूल बातें:

☐ Problem getting dressed तैयार होने में दिक़्क़त

☐ How to cook or get a meal खाना कैसे मंगवाना या बनाना है

☐ How to pay a bill बिल कैसे भरना है

**What did I have problems with? मुझे किन बातों से तकलीफ़ें हैं?**

_____

☐ I had memory problems but I don't remember what they were मुझे याददाश्त से सम्बंधित तकलीफ़ें हैं लेकिन मुझे याद नहि वे क्या थीं?

Notes: नोट्स _____

_____

## Am I Taking Care of my Brain Health?
## क्या में अपने मानसिक स्वास्थ्य का ख़याल रख रहा/रही हूँ?
## A 10-Week Journal
## १०-साप्ताहिक पत्रिका

Week [सप्ताह]: ☐ 1  ☐ 2  ☐ 3  ☐ 4  ☐ 5  ☐ 6  ☐ 7  ☐ 8  ☐ 9  ☐ 10

Today's date is [आज की तारीख़ है]:

_____

☐ Monday [सोमवार]  ☐ Tuesday [मंगलवार]  ☐ Wednesday [बुधवार]

☐ Thursday [गुरुवार]  ☐ Friday [शुक्रवार]  ☐ Saturday[शनिवार]

☐ Sunday[रविवार]

Big and small activities of the week or day: [सप्ताह या दिन के बड़े और छोटे कार्य]:

---

## Keeping Track of Healthy Brain Activities
## स्वस्थ मानसिक स्वास्थ्य पर ध्यान देना

**Brain Health** [मानसिक स्वस्थता]:

☐ **Today I** [आज में]:  ☐ **This week I**[इस हफ़्ते में]:

1. Drank enough water and made sure I was hydrated? [पर्याप्त पानी पिया और ध्यान रखा कि में जलिभूत रहूँ? ]

☐ Yes[हाँ]   ☐ No [ना]   ☐ Maybe/Somewhat [हो सकता है/कुछ हद तक]

2. Ate healthy?  [स्वास्थ्यवर्धक खाया?]

☐ Yes[हाँ]   ☐ No[ना]   ☐ Maybe/Somewhat [हो सकता है/ कुछ हद तक]

---

3. Took my medication and/or vitamins for the day? मेरी दवाई लीं और/या दिन के विटामिन लिए?

☐ Yes[हाँ]      ☐ No[ना]      ☐ Maybe/Somewhat [हो सकता है/ कुछ हद तक]

4. Had enough / good sleep last night? कल रात पर्याप्त/अच्छे से नींद ली?

☐ Yes[हाँ]      ☐ No[ना]      ☐ Maybe/Somewhat [हो सकता है/ कुछ हद तक]

5. Had stress? तनाव रहा?

☐ Yes[हाँ]      ☐ No[ना]      ☐ Maybe/Somewhat [हो सकता है/ कुछ हद तक]

Managed the stress well? तनाव को अच्छे से सम्भाला?

☐ Yes[हाँ]      ☐ No[ना]      ☐ Maybe/Somewhat [हो सकता है/ कुछ हद तक]

6. Did body exercise (walk, aerobics, etc.)? क्या शारीरिक व्यायाम किया (पैदल चलना, एरोबिक्स, आदि।)?

☐ Yes[हाँ]      ☐ No[ना]      ☐ Maybe/Somewhat [हो सकता है/ कुछ हद तक]

7. Had some kind of brain exercise? किसी तरह का मानसिक व्यायाम किया?

☐ Yes[हाँ]      ☐ No[ना]      ☐ Maybe/Somewhat [हो सकता है/ कुछ हद तक]

8. Had social time / time with family or friends? परिवार या दोस्तों के साथ सामाजिक समय बिताया?

☐ Yes[हाँ]      ☐ No[ना]      ☐ Maybe/Somewhat [हो सकता है/ कुछ हद तक]

9. Other ways to take care of brain health? अन्य तरीक़े मानसिक स्वास्थ्य का ध्यान रखने के लिए?_____

☐ Yes[हाँ]      ☐ No[ना]      ☐ Maybe/Somewhat [हो सकता है/ कुछ हद तक]

10. Other ways to take care of brain health? अन्य तरीक़े मानसिक स्वास्थ्य का ख़याल रखने के लिए?_____

☐ Yes [हाँ]      ☐ No[ना]      ☐ Maybe/Somewhat [हो सकता है/ कुछ हद तक]

Notes: नोट्स _____

_____

# Sources

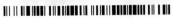

Printed in the United States
By Bookmasters